# Immunotics

Carol Colman
Robert Rountree, M.D.

# Immunotics

A Revolutionary
Way to Fight
Infection,
Beat Chronic Illness,
and Stay Well

G. P. Putnam's Sons
New York

G. P. Putnam's Sons
*Publishers Since 1838*
a member of
Penguin Putnam Inc.
375 Hudson Street
New York, NY 10014

Library of Congress Cataloging-in-Publication Data

Colman, Carol.
    Immunotics : a revolutionary way to fight infection,
    beat chronic illness, and stay well / Carol Colman and
    Robert Rountree.
        p.   cm.
    Includes bibliographical references and index.
    ISBN 0-399-14504-4
    1. Natural immunity.   2. Dietary supplements.   3. Health.
I. Rountree, Robert.   II. Title.
QR185.2.C65      2000                    00-023092
616.07′9—dc21

Printed in the United States of America

10   9   8   7   6   5   4   3   2   1

This book is printed on acid-free paper. ∞

BOOK DESIGN BY RENATO STANISIC

# Acknowledgments

I want to thank the dedicated practitioners and staff at Helios Health Center for all your help over the years. You are the best! I also want to acknowledge Jeffrey Bland, Ph.D., and the amazing group of clinicians and researchers at the Institute for Functional Medicine for being an endless source of inspiration. Your work continues to blaze the way for those of us trying to practice progressive, integrative medicine out in the "trenches." Thanks also to Aristo Vojdani, Ph.D., of Immunosciences Lab for all of his insights regarding nutritional influences on natural killer cell function. And a special thanks goes to Debbie Roth for helping me give shape to my ideas and her feedback on the manuscript.

Much thanks to my editor, Jeremy Katz, for his terrific support and input; Asha Punnett for her help; and Lori Akiyama and Cathy Fox of Penguin Putnam. A special thanks to our agent, Richard Curtis. Finally, to Carol Colman, a wonderful, brilliant partner with whom to share this project. It's been a pleasure!

# Contents

# ONE

# The Immunotics Revolution

- Do you feel like you're locked in an endless battle with every cold, flu, sinus infection, and stomach bug that comes your way?
- Does it take two to three different antibiotics to treat common infections that were once cured with just one antibiotic—or even without antibiotics at all?
- Do you have school-aged children who are plagued with chronic ear infections or sore throats?
- Do you feel that no matter what you and your family do, you can't seem to get well or stay well?
- Do you work in an office where when one person

gets sick, *everybody* gets sick? But somehow, *you* always wind up the sickest and stay sick the longest?

● Do you feel that with each passing year, you are succumbing faster and harder to common ailments that you were once able to shake off in a matter of days? Are you worried that if this downward spiral continues, you won't be able to fight off a more serious health threat, like cancer?

● Do you worry that your immune system isn't up to snuff, making you fear for the future?

If you answered yes to one or more of these questions, if you are worried that you are losing your resistance against disease, if you are sick of being sick, the Immunotics program is the answer. If you want to reclaim your health and the health of your family, if you want to fight infections, cure chronic illness, prevent disease, and *stay well*, you will find the answers you need within the pages of this book.

Immunotics is a term I have coined to describe a paradigm-changing approach to preventing and treating disease. Immunotics are to the twenty-first century what antibiotics were to the twentieth century—*but better*. Unlike antibiotics, which we use to treat illness *after* it occurs, the Immunotics program is designed to treat infections and *prevent* illness in the first place. Unlike antibiotics, which can have serious side effects, the Immunotics program has virtually none. In short, Immunotics is for anyone who refuses to accept illness as an inevitable part of life—for those who want to do everything within their power to get well and stay that way . . . safely and naturally.

Immunotics can help people of all ages—from the very

young to the very old—and at all stages of life and health. It will be particularly helpful to parents of small children who are constantly exposed to colds and other illnesses at school and bring them home to other family members. Immunotics serves people in midlife who can't bounce back from colds and flus as quickly as they used to, and will be a true lifesaver for older adults who are particularly vulnerable to common infections that younger folks can easily shake off. But Immunotics goes far beyond preventing and treating infectious disease. This revolution in health care can fortify you against other major health risks, such as cancer, which can prey on us when we are most vulnerable.

The key to the Immunotics program lies in your body's most potent weapon against disease—your immune system. Immunotics strengthens the immune system, helping it the way a computer helps our brains. Just as no computer can replace the brain, no disease fighter could ever hope to match up to the immune system. Even better, Immunotics has been specifically designed by nature to help the immune system do what it does better than anything else. We can't just replace it with antibiotics. This is a realization that is long overdue.

## Antibiotics—A Squandered Gift

Antibiotics have saved and extended millions of lives—that is undisputable. There is no better way to treat bacterial pneumonia or a nasty strep infection. When I encounter a serious medical condition that should be treated with an antibiotic, I write out a prescription in a heartbeat. I believe that antibiotics are wonderful drugs when used appropriately. Many of us wouldn't even be here without them!

Before the discovery of antibiotics, death from infection was commonplace. Rare was the family that had not seen at least one member succumb. This is still the reality in many parts of the world; I have seen it firsthand. In 1994, I worked as a volunteer physician in Ghana, where I treated hundreds of patients in remote villages. I saw children become seriously ill from virulent infections such as measles, malaria, and cholera—infections that we have eradicated in the West, thanks to antibiotics and vaccines. Antibiotics can be true lifesavers.

However, there is a dark side to these wonder drugs. As a result of their being misused, new generations of disease strains resistant to antibiotic attack have emerged. If we are not careful, within a short time, we will find ourselves back in the days when even the simplest infection could turn lethal, when death from infections in childbirth was commonplace, when tuberculosis was rampant . . . and there would be little we could do about it.

At the turn of the twentieth century, infection was the leading cause of death in the Western world, as it still is in the world at large. Thanks to the discovery of penicillin in 1928 and the introduction of other potent antibiotics in the years that followed, many infections that were usually lethal—such as tuberculosis, pneumonia, and staph—could be cured by these "magic bullets." Antibiotics seemed so miraculous that physicians and patients alike came to view them as the cure for every condition, serious or not. Have a sore throat? Take penicillin. Does the baby have an ear infection? Give her amoxicillin. Have a nasty cough and cold? Take erythromycin. Patients grew so accustomed to taking antibiotics that they demanded them routinely—whether their condition would actually respond to antibiotic therapy or not. The old-fashioned cures for colds and viruses—bed rest, warm drinks, good nutrition, and other tried and true home remedies—were considered passé. It did not matter that antibiotics are useless (and even harmful) against viruses. Patients begged for them, and doctors gave in. After all, these drugs were so great, what harm could they do? To meet this insatiable demand, pharmaceutical companies responded by flooding the market with new and stronger antibiotics.

Everyone breathed a sigh of relief. We had won the war on infection. The bugs were driven into hiding—so we thought. But they weren't defeated at all. Like a guerilla army that grows more fearsome after it is driven to the hills, the bugs started coming back. In isolated skirmishes they tested the antibiotics and found the weak points. The bugs developed new and more powerful weapons, and now it is we who are on the defensive.

What happened?

Using antibiotics to treat low-grade infections is tantamount to using a nuclear warhead to quash the schoolyard bully. It is overkill to the nth degree, yet it doesn't get rid of the problem. Just like there's always another bully hiding around the corner, there's always another strain of bacteria ready to pounce when we least expect it. Antibiotics are not foolproof—they kill most but not all of the offending bacteria. The strongest of the bacteria survive and reproduce at exponential proportions, and soon, "smart" strains of bacteria immune to the antibiotic are flourishing. The stronger the antibiotic, the stronger the surviving bacteria. To make matters worse, countless numbers of Americans have misused antibiotics by not taking the full course, stopping their medication as soon as they feel better. In so doing, they have helped create new and more powerful superbugs. Americans also use—or rather overuse—antibacterial soaps and skin products, going so far as to put antibacterial additives in toys! We are ensuring that only the hardiest of the most lethal bacteria survive. Even if you only take them when necessary and never abuse them, you may consume antibiotics without even knowing it. Around 30 percent of the antibiotics sold in the United States are fed to livestock and find their way into the meat and dairy products we eat, as well as water and soil we depend on. Think about it: Every time you eat a piece of meat or drink a glass of milk, you could be ingesting antibiotic residue, albeit in minute quantities. A genetic engineering program designed to create the ultimate germ couldn't have done any better.

## Smarter Bugs

The overuse of antibiotics over five decades has created a new breed of smarter and more virulent bacteria that are practically indestructible. For example, *Streptococcus pneumoniae*—the most common cause of bacterial ear infections in young children—has grown resistant to standard doses of amoxicillin, the first-line treatment. Drug-resistant staph infections—once easily cured with penicillin—run rampant throughout the nation's hospitals. Even more frightening is the recent discovery of staph bacteria that are resistant to vancomycin, the most powerful antibiotic on the planet! In 1941, a typical case of pneumonia could be cured with 40,000 units of penicillin a day for only four days. By 1992, pneumonia strains had grown so antibiotic resistant that a patient could receive 24 million units of penicillin a day and still die. As a recent report on antimicrobial resistance by the U. S. General Accounting Office notes, "Data indicate that resistant bacteria are emerging around the world, that more kinds of bacteria are becoming drug resistant, and that bacteria are becoming resistant to multiple drugs."

Moreover, as effective as antibiotics have been in fighting bacterial infections, bacterial infections are not the only—nor today even the greatest—threat to our health. Many infections—including those that are responsible for the common cold, AIDS, and even some forms of cancer—are caused by viruses. Viruses, which are immune to conventional antibiotics, are exceptionally difficult to defeat because they mutate rapidly, and some, such as the virus that causes AIDS, can knock out the body's ability to fight them.

These new disease strains do not respect national borders. Air travel has made it possible for an infectious disease to spread across the globe in less than a day. Modern construction practices, such as the design of windowless buildings that rely on central ventilation systems, allow bugs to spread rapidly throughout office buildings and hotels.

We are all at risk of contracting serious infections. If you fly on airplanes, work in a modern "closed" building, take care of sick children or elderly relatives, or visit friends in the hospital, your risk is enhanced. From a physician's perspective, it is frightening to have to prescribe several antibiotics to treat an infection that not too long ago would have responded to one antibiotic. I can't help but wonder, what if there comes a time when these drugs simply stop working? Experts agree that if the situation is not controlled, antibiotics will no longer work when we really need them and when our lives depend on them. In 1998, the Centers for Disease Control (CDC) in Atlanta urged physicians to start prescribing antibiotics "prudently," that is, only when absolutely necessary. In fact, according to the CDC, some *50 million* unnecessary prescriptions are written for antibiotics each year. A particularly alarming study published in the *Journal of the American Medical Association* found that doctors were routinely prescribing antibiotics for colds, bronchitis, and upper respiratory infections even though 90 percent of the time the cause was viral. The situation is so serious that some lawmakers in my home state of Colorado have even proposed legislation to make overprescription of antibiotics a crime! And a British special commission studying the problem of antibiotic resistance recently warned that "there is a dire prospect of returning to the pre-antibiotic era."

In a sense, this has already happened. More than 1 million new cases of bacterial infection occur each day, according to the World Health Organization, and most of them are drug resistant. Every year, tuberculosis, cholera, and gastrointestinal diseases that are already antibiotic resistant kill millions. According to the U. S. General Accounting Office, in 1997, hospitals discharged 43,000 patients who had been diagnosed with and treated for infections from drug-resistant bacteria.

I'm not trying to scare you. The risk of being wiped out by a virulent infection is slight, and the chance that you'll die of an antibiotic-resistant strain of bacteria is slim. Nonetheless, there are subtle, insidious costs to the overuse of antibiotics that affect us all.

Have you ever noticed how you often relapse into illness immediately after taking an antibiotic? It's not your imagination. Antibiotics can actually *weaken* your immune system, leaving you more vulnerable to the next bug that comes your way. Taking an antibiotic for common ailments that can heal on their own is particularly bad for children. What many parents may not realize is that the immune system learns through experience: Each encounter with a troublesome bacteria or virus teaches immune cells valuable lessons that will be used the next time they meet up with the same bug. Children given antibiotics for every sniffle may be robbed of their ability to effectively fight infection on their own. Yes, it may take a day or two longer for children to beat an infection without an antibiotic, but in the long run, it may be far better for the child.

Antibiotics weaken our immune system in another important way that affects both children and adults: These powerful drugs just don't kill the bad bacteria that make us sick, they also target the billions of friendly bacteria that keep us well. Without these friendly bacteria, we can't digest our food properly or keep our other systems running well. The side effects of antibiotics are not confined to a little indigestion. Antibiotics wipe out the good bacteria that keep us from getting overwhelmed by harmful E. coli infections, salmonella, and staph. Overuse of antibiotics has resulted in an epidemic of yeast infections in women. Many strains of yeast are now drug resistant, too.

Antibiotics are not bad drugs—quite the opposite—but their overuse is bad. I am a conventionally trained physician who has prescribed antibiotics for more than 20 years. But I have always tried to do so cautiously. I have spent as much time explaining to patients the correct way to take antibiotics as I have had in trying to talk them out of taking them! From my earliest days in practice, I have tried to find natural, scientifically proven alternatives to antibiotics whenever possible, and this book is the culmination of that effort. Ten years ago, I was considered avant-garde, but today, most of my colleagues have come around to my way of thinking.

## New Focus on the Immune System

The inability of antibiotics to wipe out disease entirely—and the emergence of antibiotic-resistant bacteria and superinfections—has led many distinguished researchers and physicians to conclude that the answer to disease is not to create stronger medicines. Rather, we say, the solution lies in attacking disease from the inside out, by strengthening the body's own natural defense network: the immune system. When your immune system functions well, it can usually take care of little problems before they become big ones. Every sniffle does not turn into a cold, every cold does not turn into the flu, and every flu does not turn into bronchitis. When your immune system is strong, even serious problems get nipped in the bud. Cancer cells get wiped out before they do mischief, and a little food poisoning goes almost unnoticed.

Over the past decade, scientists have learned a great deal about this remarkable system, and they have discovered new and effective ways to enhance and safeguard it. Practicing physicians like myself have taken this knowledge and put it to work, perfecting treatments to get our patients better and keep them that way. Immunotics is the science of supporting and strengthening the immune system so that it can fend off disease quickly, battle chronic illness effectively, and keep you well indefinitely. It is what I do in my medical practice every day.

This book introduces you to my easy-to-follow Immunotics program. I will show you how to combine diet, lifestyle changes, and an amazing new generation of compounds to strengthen immune function and improve your overall health and resistance to disease.

Immunotics emerged from cutting-edge science performed at laboratories around the world and two decades of clinical experience with thousands of patients. Furthermore, although I have written this book primarily for laypeople, I feel it can also be of great value to physicians. This book can, I hope, spread the word. Many conventionally trained physicians are unaware that there are simple and safe measures they can turn to when antibiotics are not warranted. They are being urged to cut back on prescriptions for antibiotics, but no one is telling them what to do instead. Immunotics provides physicians with important information that can make a real difference in the quality of life for their patients. Physicians who are curious about the science behind Immunotics or who want to do more research on it can read the bibliography at the end of this book.

## An Education by Convention, A Passion for Herbs

Before I tell you about the Immunotics program, let me tell you a bit more about my background.

I grew up in a conservative North Carolina environment where authority in general and doctors in particular were never questioned. Raised during the post–World War II baby boom when penicillin and other wonder drugs were dispensed for nearly every ailment, I, like so many others of my generation, was practically weaned on antibiotics. If you got sick, you took an antibiotic, no questions asked. Medicine meant prescribing *something*. It was as simple as that.

As a child, I never thought much about medicine. My passion was nature. I spent as much time as I could outdoors hiking and camping; for that matter, I still do. I learned to recognize many different plants, and I discovered the magic of the life processes.

Nonetheless, I was still a teenager with much to learn, and some lessons came harder than others. One particularly important lesson has shaped the way I practice medicine today. When I was a senior in high school, I began to suffer from terrible respiratory symptoms, including a chronic, wheezing cough. Amazingly, I did not attribute these symptoms to the fact that I smoked two packs of cigarettes a day, but what was even more amazing was neither did the allergist I consulted! His advice was to eliminate 30 common foods from my diet and to get weekly allergy injections. Skeptical of his diagnosis, I spotted a pack of cigarettes in the doctor's pocket, and it suddenly dawned on me that maybe my problems had more to do with the two packs of cigarettes daily I was inhaling directly into my lungs than food allergies. I stopped smoking and started reading books about health. I made some modest changes in my diet to include more fruits and vegetables and less junk food. I began taking vitamins. Within a few months, the cough had vanished and my chest was clear. I had found the "cure" simply by giving my body the tools it needed to repair itself. After this experience, safeguarding my own health became second nature to me. It is a lesson I have tried to pass on to the thousands of patients who have been in my care.

At the University of North Carolina, I continued my study

of the life sciences and would have become a biologist had I not stumbled on a book that was to change the direction of my life: *Herbs: The Magic Healers,* by Paul Twitchell. That review of herbal medicine as it was practiced around the world included many of the same plants I had identified in the North Carolina woods as a boy! Intrigued by the book, I ventured into a local herb shop. Today, herbs are sold in pristine bottles and blister packs in mainstream drugstores, pharmacies, and health food stores. Back then, herbs were only sold in bulk out of huge wooden barrels under primitive conditions. You really didn't know what you were buying, much less how to use them. The only references were old-fashioned herbals (some written hundreds of years ago) that contained much folklore and anecdotes but little science. I learned that echinacea had been used for centuries to treat colds and flus, but no one knew that it worked by boosting the immune system. I read that goldenseal was a natural antibiotic, but few agreed on how to use it. I found myself fascinated by the healing power of the natural world, and I decided to explore it. But I was already a scientist (in a sense I always had been) and I needed to better understand how herbs and other natural healing agents worked.

I attended medical school at the University of North Carolina at Chapel Hill and did my residency in family medicine at the Milton S. Hershey Medical Center in Hershey, Pennsylvania. I surprised my teachers and peers by choosing to pursue a general family practice as opposed to a more "prestigious" specialty, but I had never doubted that I would be a family practitioner. It was the only specialty that allowed me to treat the entire patient, not one small part of the body. It introduced me to entire families, from the youngest infants to the oldest of the old and everyone in between, and provided the ideal environment to develop my brand of integrative medicine: the merging of natural medicine with good science.

After my residency, I became a family practice physician in Boulder, where I cofounded Helios Health Center in 1993. Now, I'm proud to say, the center is thriving. We are the primary physicians for thousands of patients and treat every kind of medical problem imaginable. In practice, I've continued my love and study of the natural world and its healing powers, and over the years I've developed an impressive arsenal of alternative methods to treat common ailments safely and effectively. My Immunotics program is based on this experience and passion of a lifetime.

## The Immunotics Program

The Immunotics program mounts a four-pronged attack against disease:

- The Immunotics Pharmacy
- The Immunotics Food Plan
- Your Mind: A Powerful Immunotic
- Creating An Immune-Friendly Environment

### The Immunotics Pharmacy

This book will introduce you to tried and true "immunotics"—supplements to bolster immune function and treat disease. In chapter 4, I review the 30 extraordinary immunotics that form the foundation of the program. Everything that I recommend is available over the counter at neighborhood health food stores, pharmacies, discount stores, and even supermarkets. Here are some highlights.

*Colostrum:* Why do breast-fed infants get sick less often than bottle-fed infants? Breast milk contains powerful immune-bolstering proteins that help keep infants well throughout their first months of life. A protein derived from the first milk produced by a nursing mother, colostrum is a rich source of these immune-stimulating compounds. For the rest of us, bovine colostrum, available in powder and capsules, is an excellent general immune booster, especially for people with chronic infections. It is as safe as mother's milk!

*Olive leaf extract:* Many of you know that olive oil is good for your health, but what you may not know is that an extract derived from the leaf of the olive is a potent natural antibiotic and antiviral. It also gives the immune system a much-needed boost. It is a terrific treatment for acute infections, such as sore throats and bad colds. When my patients beg for an antibiotic (and I know it won't help them) I prescribe olive leaf extract. It helps them beat the infection faster—with no side effects.

*NAC:* Long used in hospitals to treat acetaminophen overdose and cystic fibrosis, NAC is now sold over the counter. My first-line treatment for upper-respiratory infections, it is particularly good at clearing up a congested nose.

*Garlic:* Garlic has been used for thousands of years in traditional medicine as an effective treatment for stomach bugs. Garlic can be eaten raw (I explain how in chapter 4) or taken in capsule form.

*Western larch:* I prescribe this herb, available in a powder form that can be mixed in juice, for nasty ear infections or bad colds in children. It is a safe, inexpensive, and easy-to-use immune booster that gives the body added ammunition to fight off infection.

Chapter 6 provides a basic Immunotics supplement program designed to enhance overall immune function. In addition to the Basic Immunotics Program, this chapter contains modified programs for readers with special risk factors and vulnerabilities. For example, if you seem to catch every cold that comes your way, follow the program designed to fortify your immune system against respiratory problems. If you tend to come down with stomach bugs, I'll show you how to protect yourself against digestive disorders. If you are at high risk of developing cancer, try the program designed to boost your cancer-fighting immune cells.

But under the best of circumstances, even the healthiest people get sick. In chapter 7, I will show you how to use immunotics to relieve symptoms and speed recovery from common illnesses such as low-grade infections, sore throats, ear infections, respiratory ailments, and others. I will also tell you how immunotics can be useful as an adjuvant treatment for more serious problems such as cancer, AIDS, and hepatitis.

## The Immunotics Food Plan

As good as immunotics supplements may be, they are meant to work in synergy with food, not as a substitute for good nutrition. Food is a wonderful source of natural immunotics, but unfortunately, few people take advantage of nature's food pharmacy. In fact, as you will learn in chapter 3—"Are You at Risk?"—an inadequate diet is the number one cause of poor immune function! Simply put, most of us are eating too much of the wrong foods and too little of the right ones. However, by making modest changes in your diet, you can make a huge difference in your ability to maintain optimal immune health. If you find yourself sick all too often, I strongly urge you to pay close attention to the Immunotics food plan.

Outlined in chapter 8, the Immunotics food plan shows you how easy it is to eat foods that work *with* your body to fight disease and strengthen immune function. To make things really simple, I list superfoods that you should eat every day. Even if you do nothing else than incorporate at least some of these foods into your daily diet, I guarantee you'll see a positive result.

### Your Mind: A Powerful Immunotic

Caring for your body by taking the immunotics supplements, eating wisely, and getting enough exercise is important, but it does not do the whole job of achieving optimal immune health. Clinical studies have proven that your mind—what you think and feel—has a powerful effect on your immune system. Learning how to harness that power not only can help keep you well but also will help you heal more quickly if you're not. It is every bit as important a component of the Immunotics program as supplements, nutrition, and a healthy environment. In fact, there are times when I believe that our feelings about illness and our visions of the future may be THE determining factor in whether we succumb or survive. In chapter 9, I discuss the techniques you can use to tap the power of the forgotten immunotic: the mind.

Creating an Immune-friendly Environment

Chapter 10 provides specific tips on how to create an immune-friendly lifestyle that minimizes the risk of getting sick. Simple changes in your everyday habits can demonstrably enhance immune function. In particular, this chapter will help people living in high-risk situations, such as those who work in poorly ventilated office buildings or hospitals, parents of school-aged children who are always getting sick, and frequent travelers.

## A Word to Readers

The underlying philosophy of my medical practice is that physicians first and foremost should be educators. As a physician, I am privileged to have access to information that most patients do not. It is my obligation to share that information. Twenty years of practice have taught me that my patients are intelligent and that given the right information they will make the right choices. I have written this book to share my knowledge with you so that you too can make the right choices for yourself and your family.

# TWO

# Your Immune System: Your Body's Best Weapon Against Disease

The immune system is the sole reason why we humans can live in a world vastly outnumbered by thousands of trillions of potential enemies and not only survive but thrive. Coated with protein and sugar, the human body is a feast to microscopic life—and the only thing standing between "us" and "them" is the immune system. It allows us personal space on a planet teeming with hungry microorganisms. Without it, we would be vulnerable to every bacteria, virus, fungus, and parasite that came our way.

Our immune system also protects us against invaders from within, which can be the most threatening of all. If, for example, our bodies produce a cancer cell by mistake, a vigilant immune system usually destroys it before the cancer can spread. Immune cells function as the body's bouncer, constantly on alert for troublemakers. When it is working well, the immune system is the line in the sand that tells unwanted intruders, "You can go this far, and no farther." When the line gets blurred, we get sick.

The immune system is one of the smartest systems in the body. It not only knows when to get tough but, of equal importance, it knows when to leave well enough alone. Our survival depends on its ability to distinguish friend from foe. For example, if the immune system targeted every foreign protein to enter our bodies, we would reject the food we eat before it could be digested and absorbed. If the immune system could not discern between the protein of an invading virus and a fertilized human egg cell, we could not reproduce. New life would be nipped in the bud. If the immune system was unable to distinguish between our own protein and the protein of outside invaders, immune cells would attack the very cells and organs that make up our bodies! Incidentally, that is precisely what happens in autoimmune diseases such as rheumatoid arthritis, lupus, and multiple sclerosis.

To understand the importance of the immune system—and, more important, how to keep it humming along—you need to know a bit about how it works.

First, in the interest of full disclosure, I'd like to issue this disclaimer: We do not fully understand what this system is and what makes it run, and the more we learn about it, the more we recognize the gaps in our knowledge. Nevertheless, we have a basic idea of how the immune system functions.

## Where Is the Immune System?

Everywhere. The immune system is not confined to one organ or one site in the body—it is everywhere, in every place—some of which may surprise you. The immune system is not a discrete entity, but rather an assortment of billions of specialized cells that protect the body in many different ways. The system's agents, the immune cells, occupy every part of the body—the skin, the eyes, the nostrils, the lungs, and the lining of our internal organs. There they stand guard protecting us from potential troublemakers. There are many different types of immune cells. Some immune cells circulate throughout the body, putting out fires wherever they find them. Others patrol the lining and blood vessels of particular organs. The mucus in nasal passages and other parts of the body is an important component of the immune system. It traps dust, pollen, bacteria, viruses, and pollutants from the air. The lining of the gastrointestinal (GI) tract houses a huge concentration of immune cells. That makes perfect sense; after all, the gut is continually exposed to microorganisms and toxins from our diets. Even skin is part of the immune system. It holds up the first barrier that unwanted invaders must penetrate in order to gain entrance into our bodies.

Immune cells circulate throughout the body within the lymphatic system, a separate network from the circulatory system, which transports blood throughout the body. The vessels of the lymphatic system contain lymph, a pale, thick fluid consisting of fat and white blood cells. When the immune system hears a distress call from one part of the body, it rapidly dispatches immune cells via the lymphatic system to the problem area.

The immune system includes four key organs: the lymph nodes, bone marrow, thymus gland, and spleen, which are interconnected via the lymphatic system.

*Lymph nodes.* The lymph nodes are glandlike organs found in many sites in the body, including under the arms, behind the ears, and in the groin. When we have "swollen glands," it means that our lymph nodes are inflamed and the immune system is activated. Part of the lymphatic system, lymph nodes act like drains to remove or extract foreign particles from entering the bloodstream. Think of lymph nodes as filters designed to keep harmful organisms out of the bloodstream, where they could be circulated to the major organs of the body.

*Bone marrow.* All red blood cells, including most immune cells, are produced within the bone marrow from special cells called stem cells. Once they have matured— that is, are ready for action—immune cells from bone marrow migrate to various parts of the immune system via the lymphatic system.

*Thymus.* A pinkish-gray gland that sits behind the breastbone, the thymus is another site in the body where immune cells are produced. Important immune cells called T-cells are made in the thymus and then are sent to the bone marrow to mature. The thymus weighs less than 2 ounces at birth and doubles in size by puberty. After that it begins to shrink and is replaced by fatty tissue.

*Spleen.* The spleen, a dark red, flat organ located behind the stomach, is another site where immune cells are produced. The spleen also helps cleanse the blood of unwanted invaders.

## Teamwork

The immune system consists of several different types of cells that work together to keep us healthy. A brief description follows of some of the most important immune cells and how they work. As you will see in chapter 4, "The Immunotics Pharmacy," many immunotics work by enhancing the number and/or activity level of specific immune cells.

### B-Cells: They Have Memory

Special immune cells produced in the bone marrow, B-cells are critical for normal immune function, but before you can understand what they do and why they are so valuable, you need to know more about immune cell activity. Not all immune cells do the same job. Some immune cells attack foreign proteins (antigens) at random as they enter the body. This system is not foolproof—these trigger-happy immune cells do not always get their antigens. But the immune system is sophisticated enough to compensate for this problem and actually to plan for it. If an antigen is not quickly destroyed by the first line of defense, there is plenty of backup. Here's where the B-cells show their stuff—if they encounter an antigen, they "tag" the invader with proteins called antibodies (or immunoglobulins), which alert other immune cells of imminent danger. The antibody tag is critical for our defense; in fact, many immune cells will not attack an antigen unless it has an antibody tag.

B-cells have good memories. Once an antibody is produced against an antigen, the immune system is forever on guard against that particular antigen. If the same antigen should try to attack again, it will be quickly recognized and destroyed before it can do harm. That is why once you get chicken pox or measles, you don't get it again—your body is ready to pounce the minute it reappears.

Vaccination is an ingenious way of using B-cells to create immunity. A vaccine is a weakened or killed strain of a virus or a disease-causing bacteria or a fragment of that virus or bacteria. Although it is not strong enough to make you sick, the vaccine will stimulate your B-cells to produce antibodies so that when you encounter the same infection, you are already protected. Potentially deadly diseases such as polio, tetanus, whooping cough, and smallpox have been almost eradicated, thanks to vaccines.

Antibodies are Y-shaped molecules. The "V" portion binds to the foreign proteins and varies from antibody to antibody. There are literally thousands of possible variations. However, the bottom portion of the antibody forms a chemical structure that is identical to other similar antibodies in the same group. There are only five permutations; thus antibodies are classified into five groups: IgA, IgG, IgM, IgE, and IgD.

IgA is the first step in alerting the immune system of an imminent invasion. It is the primary antibody that is released in the walls of the mucus membranes and the cells that line the intestinal tract, two particularly vulnerable points in the body. A healthy person produces up to 10 grams of secretory IgA daily, a huge amount. Mother's milk, particularly colostrum, is extremely high in IgA.

IgM is the antibody that is produced after initial exposure

to an antigen. For example, after receiving a measles vaccination, levels of IgM rise within 10 to 14 days.

IgG is the most prevalent type of antibody. It is called into action after IgM does its job. Once the immune system is familiar with the newly identified enemy—thanks to IgM—subsequent IgG antibody production is faster and more abundant. IgG is transferred across the placenta from the mother to the fetus, protecting the fetus and newborn from disease.

IgE is the antibody involved in allergic reactions; it helps the body reject substances such as excess dust. If IgE becomes overzealous, however, it could trigger allergic reactions to normally benign substances such as pollen and dust mites. IgE stimulates special cells called mast cells to release histamine, a chemical that is important for digestion and the dilation of small blood vessels but that in excess can cause allergic symptoms. Levels of IgE are very high in people with chronic parasitic infection (such as roundworm), which is why scientists believe this antibody must protect against parasites.

IgD is the antibody found in small amounts in circulating blood, but its function is not fully understood.

### Natural Killer Cells

B-cells attack antigens indirectly by producing antibodies, leaving the hand-to-hand combat to other cells, such as natural killer—or NK—cells, a type of small white blood cell (or lymphocyte). While there are several different types of lymphocytes, each with a very specific job, between 5 and 15 percent of them are NK cells. NK cells are critical for our survival. Unique among immune cells, NK cells are not summoned into action by an antibody; rather, they have the innate ability to attack an intruder on their own.

NK cells have many different functions in the immune system, but primarily they deal with controlling cancer cells and acute infection. For example, when the body is challenged by a new virus, bacteria, or cancerous cell, an army of NK cells wage the first assault. NK cells can produce a substance called interferon, which prevents viruses from replicating. They also release poisonous chemicals such as nitric oxide that destroy the internal machinery of the invading cell.

I can't overestimate the importance of NK cells. NK activity—the ability of NK cells to detect and attack the body's enemies—is an excellent barometer of overall health and can be measured by a simple blood test that is performed at a diagnostic laboratory. I often recommend the test for my patients with cancer or a strong family history of cancer, and for good reason, too: People with a high family incidence of cancer often have low NK cell activity. Not surprisingly, studies have shown that people with active NK cells are the least likely to get sick, while people with sluggish NK cells are the most vulnerable. They are less likely to beat a serious illness like cancer.

NK cells appear to play a pivotal role in the spread of cancer. Patients with metastatic breast cancer or metastatic melanoma (meaning the disease has spread to other organs) have lower NK cell activity than patients whose cancers have stayed confined to one site. In fact, NK activity in cancer patients is often a predictor of whether a patient will survive or succumb to the disease. Sluggish NK cells have also been linked to chronic fatigue syndrome. Does the fact that you may have been born with low NK cell activity—or may develop it sometime in your life—mean that you are condemned to illness? Not at all! Fortunately, we know of several effective ways to boost NK cell activity, including several of the immunotics supplements I recommend. I have seen patients on immunotics double their NK activity often within a few weeks. They do better on their lab tests and demonstrate improved health.

NK cells also produce hormonelike chemicals called cytokines, which are the mechanism by which immune cells communicate. Cytokines regulate some of the activities of other immune cells.

Interestingly, a link joins low NK cell activity with the ability to handle emotional stress. In fact, chronic stress can dampen NK cell activity, while relaxation exercises such as meditation can enhance it. I'll explain more about the fascinating connection between stress and immunity in chapter 9.

### Neutrophils: The Workhorses

Neutrophils are the main circulating white blood cells of the immune system. They travel through the bloodstream searching out potential troublemakers and pay special attention to bacteria. When people have bacterial infection, their levels of neutrophils typically are elevated. Neutrophils are not particularly "smart"—that is, they do not recognize and seek out specific microorganisms—but if they should encounter "bad" bacteria, they engulf and destroy it. Like NK cells, neutrophils produce toxins that kill antigens and then ingest them. Unlike NK cells, which are autonomous, neutrophils are summoned into action by other immune cells.

## Macrophages: The "Big Eaters"

Macrophages are large cells residing in the organs that directly interface with the bloodstream or come into contact with the outside world (such as the liver, which connects to blood vessels, and the lungs, which inhale air). Similar to neutrophils, macrophages devour foreign material, but unlike their ubiquitous cousins, some of them do not circulate freely in the bloodstream—they stay put and protect the specific area to which they have been assigned. Think of macrophages as the garbage collectors of the immune system. Macrophages in the lungs help "digest" inhaled dust and other toxins. The macrophages found in the bone marrow, connective tissue, and lining of major organs perform similar tasks. While they tend to be homebodies, when a part of the body becomes infected, macrophages rush to the point of infection. They work in tandem with neutrophils, attracting their junior partners to the problem area to help gobble up the bad stuff. Macrophages also release a substance called pyrogen that signals the body to raise its temperature to cook the offending virus or bacteria.

## T Is for Thymus

T-lymphocytes are white blood cells produced in the thymus, hence the name T-cells. T-cells fight against cancer and certain types of bacterial, viral, and fungal infections. While T-cells don't produce antibodies, they work in tandem with the cells that do. Like NK cells and neutrophils, T-cells circulate throughout the body looking for potential trouble, but unlike these other immune cells, T-cells do not attack at random. Rather, T-cells look for the antibody tag before attacking a specific invader.

All T-cells are not the same.

- Cytotoxic T-cells race to the site of invasion and attach themselves to the troublemakers.
- Helper T-cells (also known as T4 or CD4 cells) stimulate B-lymphocytes to produce antibodies. There are two kinds of helper T-cells; T-helper 1 and T-helper 2. T-helper 1 cells primarily fight infection, while T-helper 2 cells are mainly involved in allergic and inflammatory responses. When they are behaving normally, T-helper 2 cells protect the body from dust and other unwanted substances, but if these cells become overactive, they can trigger allergic reactions to proteins that pose no threat to the body (such as pollen, food substances, etc.)
- Suppressor T-cells tell the B-lymphocytes when enough antibodies have been produced and tell the cytotoxic T-cells to retreat.

At one time it was believed that autoimmune diseases were caused by an excess of helper cells and a deficiency in suppressor cells. Scientists now believe that this explanation is simplistic and suspect that in some people, an imbalance of T-helper 1 cells and T-helper 2 cells could be the trigger that sends the immune system into overdrive. To be honest, no one knows for sure, and when it comes to these diseases, there are no easy answers. People with lupus have different immune responses from people with rheumatoid arthritis. When it comes to understanding the mechanisms of the immune system, the more we learn, the more we realize what we don't know.

The importance of T-cells is brought into focus by the AIDS epidemic. HIV is so deadly because it specifically targets and attacks T-cells. Over time, the growing lack of T-cells weakens the immune system. In other words, you don't die from AIDS: you die from the opportunistic infections that flourish in a compromised immune system.

## The Immune System Can Learn

We tend to think that the brain is the only center of learning in the body, but that's not true. The immune system learns constantly from the first day of life to the last. In the first eight weeks of a child's life, the immune system is underdeveloped, or *immunonaive*. The little one has no real-life experience with pathogens and is often defenseless against a serious infection like strep. Its immune system hasn't learned the ropes yet. For that reason, physicians recommend that a newborn be kept in relative seclusion for up to eight weeks until the immune system can develop. Breast-feeding, however, can help the infant's immune system work better and faster. The best nourishment there is for your baby, breast milk also contains important proteins that enhance immune function. Breast milk is a vehicle through which the mother can pass her "experienced" immunity on to her "naive" infant. In particular, colostrum, the first milk produced by new mothers, is a potent source of immune-strengthening proteins—an intensive seminar for a young and inexperienced immune system. (Colostrum derived from cow's milk is one of the newest and most effective immunotics; see chapter 4.)

Vaccination is another way of jump-starting the immune system. From the age of two months on, we begin vaccinating children against the major childhood diseases such as diphtheria, tetanus, chicken pox, whooping cough, hemophilus influenza, and hepatitis. Without ever encountering the antigen in real life, the child's B-cells begin producing antibodies against it.

Vaccinations are not just for children—they also work for adults. For example, each year, millions of people take influenza vaccines to prevent the flu. You may wonder, if vaccinations work so well, why can't we develop vaccines against every potential illness, such as HIV, the virus that causes AIDS? Creating a vaccine is not as easy as it sounds. It can be very tricky to develop the right vaccine—one that is strong enough to stimulate immunity but does not cause the disease it is trying to prevent! Moreover, bacteria and viruses are very clever. They have the ability to mutate or change their genetic makeup as conditions change. Every year brings, for example, a new strain of influenza, and every year we make a new vaccine to conquer it. Finally, making a vaccine for every ailment on earth is not practical. The common cold alone boosts more than two hundred different viruses. You can't vaccinate against everything. You still need to rely on your immune system to protect you against the vast majority of illnesses.

## Immune Cells Talk to One Another

I noted earlier that the immune system is smart, but until recently I don't think we fully appreciated just how smart it is. Similar to the way nerve cells talk to one another via a network of chemicals called neurotransmitters, the cells of the immune system have their own method of communication. Immune cells produce hormonelike substances called cytokines, which transmit information to other immune cells. Immune cells "listen" to cytokines and can recognize subtle changes in cytokine production, which can then trigger an immune response. Macrophages summon neutrophils via cytokines; NK cells mobilize T-cells by sending out cytokines. Not only can cytokines communicate with immune cells but a particular type of cytokine, called interleukins, talk to nerve cells, thereby creating a link between the immune system and the nervous system. This raises an interesting point. In recent years, we've heard a great deal about the body/mind connection in medicine, and most of the research in this area has centered on the role the brain plays in controlling health. In fact, when I was describing NK cell activity, I noted that stress can dampen NK function. The underlying assumption of body/mind research has always been that the brain is the dominant player that controls the immune system. For example, cancer patients who join support groups often live longer than those who don't, suggesting that social support can influence physical health. We also know that it is possible to measurably enhance immune function through visualization techniques in which a patient imagines a scenario in which "good" immune cells attack "bad" cancer cells. But we're learning that the mind/body connection is not a one-way street. The latest research on interleukins suggest that the immune system does not passively listen to the brain. Instead, there is a feedback mechanism between the two. For example, it's very common for people with bad colds to become emotionally overwrought. I have seen people with nasty colds start weeping for no apparent reason. At first glance, this appears to be an extreme reaction to a mild and curable condition, but given what we now know about cytokines, I think it goes deeper. When you have a cold, your immune system is suddenly kicked into high gear. Your immune cells are pumping out more cytokines, telling the brain, "Hey, we're under attack." The brain processes this information by becoming upset and anxious. I have come to the conclusion that our personality and behavior on a day-to-day basis is profoundly influenced by what our immune system is doing—and saying—to our brains. The brain/immune system connection has been a particular interest of mine and one I have pursued with my patients. I describe some of the behaviorial techniques I use to support immune function in chapter 9.

## Bacteria: Friends and Enemies of the Immune System

The immune system is activated when it discovers a potentially harmful microorganism, such as a troublesome bacteria that could trigger an ear infection or cause a sore throat. Bacteria are primitive, single-celled organisms that are classified according to their shape. Spherical bacteria are known as cocci (i.e., the streptococcus causes strep throat); rodlike bacteria as bacilli, spiral-shaped bacteria as spirillum, comma-shaped bacteria as vibrio, and corkscrew-shaped bacteria as spirochetes. There is no escaping bacteria; they are everywhere. They live in soil, water, food, air, on our skin, and within our bodies. Fortunately, not all bacteria are bad—if they were, we would have succumbed to them a long time ago. Helpful bacteria, known as probiotics, live within the gut and help with digestion and control the overgrowth of bad bacteria. In fact, studies suggest that these good bacteria may even help prevent cancer. (For more on probiotics, see chapter 4.) Even potentially harmful bacteria at low levels are harmless for most healthy people. Some scientists speculate that low-grade, ongoing exposure to these bad bugs keeps the immune system in good working order.

Despite the popular belief that bacteria are our sworn enemies, in reality, they mean us no harm—they are only looking for a nice place to reproduce. But if they reproduce too quickly or in the wrong place, they can be deadly. During reproduction, some bacteria release harmful enzymes that cause inflammation and tissue damage. It is not necessarily the bacteria that make us sick but the damage created from their reproduction. Some bacteria, such as those that cause botulism, produce toxins when they die. They can be the most poisonous of them all.

Bacteria have a proclivity for particular spots in the body. Those areas contain binding proteins that "fit" into corresponding areas on the bacteria. For example, certain bacteria congregate in the spinal fluid, causing spinal meningitis, and the ones that cause endocarditis bind to sites in the heart. Some are particularly at home in the lining of the gut, while others stick to the walls of the bladder. Some bacteria thrive in moist parts of the body, others seek out the warmest parts. If it weren't for this bacterial preference, every major infection we get would attack our entire body.

Bacteria existed long before the human race appeared on earth and will undoubtedly be around long after we're gone. Although they are a primitive form of life, they are resilient and even clever. Since the discovery of penicillin, medicine has relied on antibiotics to defeat this foe, but these enemies have often stayed ahead of us.

Our weapon against bacteria is antibiotics—drugs that destroy microbes. Some antibiotics are specific to particular bacteria, while others are broad-spectrum. Typically, antibiotics kill bacteria by attaching to a specific target site, usually the cell wall. The cell wall allows the bacteria to maintain the correct levels of fluid and nutrients—the microbial equivalent of skin. The antibiotic weakens the cell wall, allowing vital substances to leak out, thereby destroying the cell.

Bacteria have developed ingenious methods to elude antibiotics. Some bacteria defend themselves by altering the target site; then the antibiotic has no place to bind. Other bacteria have learned to produce enzymes that deactivate specific drugs. The savvy bacteria (i.e., the ones still alive) pass this information on to their descendants, creating antibiotic-resistant strains. Humans have helped in this process by misusing antibiotics. For example, people often ignore doctor's orders and stop taking an antibiotic once symptoms disappear, before they have completed the full treatment course. Although they may have taken the antibiotic long enough to kill enough of the offending bacteria to feel better, the remaining bacteria can mutate and develop a resistant strain. It's natural selection sped up a thousandfold.

## Viruses: Our Bitter Foes

Viruses are strands of genetic material—DNA or RNA—encased in a protective protein shield. Completely parasitic, they cannot exist without a host; unlike bacteria, they cannot live outside the body or reproduce on their own. They need to "borrow" the genetic machinery (the DNA or RNA) of other organisms to reproduce, so they hijack the cells of the host. The most successful viruses, like HIV, don't kill their hosts immediately but stay within the body for years at a time.

Viruses are immune to conventional antibiotics, but new antiviral drugs such as acyclovir (Zovirax) can prevent viruses from replicating. However, they can't eliminate the virus from your system. That's up to your immune system. If you are using an antiviral drug, it is essential to take it as early as possible to stop the virus from reproducing.

The immune system has an elaborate defense mechanism against viruses. Most often, it poisons them with toxic chemicals called free radicals. In what's called an oxidative burst, white blood cells release a potent form of oxygen that often destroys the virus but can also damage healthy tissue. It's not only the virus that's making you feel sick, but the immune system's response. If the immune system reacts too strongly, it could even kill you.

Some viruses, like cold viruses, are very easy to catch. Transmitted through casual contact, when someone coughs or sneezes or even shakes hands with an infected person, the virus leaps from host to host. An airborne virus can land on a doorknob or a plate, waiting to ambush the next victim who touches the infected area and then puts his hands in his mouth, nose, or eyes. Other viruses, such as HIV, are quite difficult to catch. They are transmitted through the exchange of blood from sharing needles or transfusions, the exchange of body fluids through sexual contact, or breast-feeding. Although HIV can be deadly, it is easy to avoid it by following simple precautions.

Viruses can be just as wily as bacteria, perhaps even more so. Some can lie dormant for years. Chicken pox virus, for example, lies in wait in nerve endings, resurfacing decades later as shingles. Some are ingenious. HIV knocks out T-helper cells, leaving the immune system underdefended.

And like clockwork every year, flu viruses mutate into a new and brutal strain. Don't underestimate the power of viruses. Each year the flu kills some 20,000 people, many of them with weakened immune systems. A particularly virulent one could kill millions. The very young—the immunonaive—are especially vulnerable, as are people over 65. Vaccinations against the year's flu strain are available each fall, but they are not as effective in older people as in younger people.

## Fungal Infections

Fungi are simple plants, including yeasts, that can also live within our bodies. An overgrowth of a particular type of fungus, candida albicans (and related candida species) is responsible for vaginal yeast infections in women. Fungi are usually controlled by "good" bacteria that live in the gut, but they can easily get out of control. Fungi thrive in the warm, moist environment of the human body; and once they settle, they are difficult to evict. NK cells and T-cells target fungi, but they don't always win, and antifungal medicines are inconsistent. Probiotics, along with immunotics that boost NK cell activity, are the best way to get rid of a troublesome fungal infection.

## The Aging Immune System

We are born with a "naive" immune system that matures over time until it is functioning at peak capacity. During childhood and young adulthood, we can shake off sniffles and minor problems with relative ease. Every cold doesn't turn into a sinus infection, and every flu doesn't put us at risk of pneumonia. Our risk of developing cancer is significantly lower than when we are older. It is easy to take our good health for granted! As we age, however, our immune system ages too, leaving us vulnerable to illnesses of all kinds. We call this stage of life immunosenescence.

Although we still have the same number of disease-fighting T-cells, they are no longer as effective as they used to be. Our NK cells grow sluggish, failing to weed out bad bacteria, viruses, and cancerous cells before they can spread. Our antibodies become "forgetful" and may not alert the immune system to potential troublemakers. The immune cells responsible for suppressing immune response may get sloppy, allowing immune cells to destroy the body's own tissue, causing autoimmune disorders.

In all likelihood, the decline in immune function is part of the general slowdown that befalls all body systems as we age. I believe, however, that it is possible to maintain a vigorous immune system well into old age. But I also believe that not taking adequate care of yourself accelerates immune decline. As you will see in chapter 3, "Are You at Risk?" poor nutrition and an unhealthy lifestyle are the two most important factors in maintaining immune health. The earlier you begin taking care of yourself the better, but it's never too late. I have seen people of all ages make dramatic progress. If you are stuck in immunosenescence, if you are fighting chronic infection, getting sick more frequently, or have been diagnosed with cancer, the Immunotics program can be of great value in helping you to regain your immune health.

# THREE

## Are You at Risk?

**N**ot all immune systems are created equal. Some people are born lucky, with the gift of good health and a hardy immune system. These few rarely get sick. Nature, however, has given most of us a less-than-perfect pedigree. Under the right (or wrong) set of circumstances, we can and will get sick. Oftentimes, we compound our vulnerabilities by neglecting, overtaxing, and ultimately weakening our immune system. In the pages that follow, I will alert you to the major risk factors in your life that may have an adverse effect on your immune system, your health, and ultimately, your life.

If there were nothing to be done, it would be pointless— and unfair—to alarm you about risk factors that could be hurting your immune health. Fortunately, that's not the case. Most of the risk factors listed here can be mitigated with the judicious use of the Immunotics program. Even risk factors that may appear to be outside of your control can be improved—and improved significantly—by taking the proper precautions. Only through understanding your personal risk factors can you turn your immune system around.

The most common reasons why your immune system may not be operating as well as it should are as follows.

## Micronutrient Starvation: The Number One Enemy of the Immune System

Micronutrient starvation is a silent foe—its harmful effects may not be felt for years, yet it is the number one cause of poor immune function and, therefore, disease.

Micronutrients include vitamins, minerals, and important chemicals found in plant foods (called phytochemicals). Some micronutrients are well known, such as vitamin C and calcium, while others may be less familiar, such as carotenoids and bioflavonoids. Even though many micronutrients may not be listed on the side of a cereal box and don't have an RDA, they are essential for optimal health. One out of four Americans is clinically obese, but despite this fact, many of us consume diets so seriously deficient in micronutrients that our bodies are literally starved for them. You can be well fed and even overweight and still be malnourished. In the end, it is your immune system that suffers.

Micronutrient starvation is not the same as having a severe vitamin deficiency disease, such as scurvy (a deficiency in vitamin C ) or beri beri (a deficiency in thiamine, a B vitamin). Both scurvy and beri beri, rare in the Western world but still common in Africa, usually result from true starvation. They can be deadly. Micronutrient starvation may not kill us right away, but over time it has a devastating impact on health.

Micronutrients abound in the fruits and vegetables we're accustomed to seeing on store shelves. Yet only 10 percent of the American population consumes the five servings of fruits and vegetables daily recommended by the National Institutes of Health. Many go through the day without eating even one serving! Move a couple of aisles over, and micronutrients become scarce in the foods typical of American cuisine. They are all but nonexistent in fast foods, overly processed foods, and junk foods. Refined sugar, found in large quantities in nearly every processed food, not only is devoid of nutrients but may *suppress* immune function. As a result, countless numbers of Americans suffer from subclinical deficiencies in key micronutrients, with untold effect on their immune function. Numerous studies have documented that when blood levels of key vitamins, minerals, and phytochemicals drop below optimal levels, our immune systems don't function properly. Numerous studies have also documented that people who eat diets richest in key micronutrients are at a substantially lower risk of developing many different diseases. The message is clear: The right micronutrients can keep you healthy.

Although I recommend that people take supplements, I believe that there is no substitute for a good diet. It's the key to good health. Period. In fact, many of the immunotics that I recommend can be found in foods you already eat (albeit in less potent form than when taken as a supplement). For example, fruits and vegetables are a terrific source of antioxidants. Another class of immunotics called beta glucans are abundant in oat bran, whole grains, and Asian mushrooms such as shiitake. Bioflavonoids, yet another important immunotic, are found in abundance in red grapes, berries, oranges, tea, and other fruits and vegetables.

Scores of other phytochemicals have been shown to have a positive effect on immune function; I go into that in depth in chapter 8. When it comes to preserving and strengthening your immune system, no magic pill can substitute for smart nutrition. Granted, when you're sick, you may need to turn to a stronger immunotic, but I believe that eating a diet rich in immune-boosting substances will reduce the odds of getting sick in the first place!

## Immunosenescence: The Aging of the Immune System

Children and teenagers amaze me. They can bounce back practically overnight after a bad cold or virus while the same ailment can send their parents to bed for days—even weeks—at a time. A young immune system hums along like a well-oiled machine, but an older immune system begins to get creaky. Like everything else in our bodies, it ages. Although no one knows precisely why it does, current thinking links declining immunity to the age-related decline in key hormones (such as DHEA) and general wear and tear. The problem begins around midlife, when people begin to notice a subtle change in their ability to resist and recover from illness. A cough that would have at one time just faded away might now spiral into a respiratory infection. A virus that would have lasted no more than 24 hours now leaves us out of commission for several days. As we age, our immune cells begin to lose some of their vim and vigor, resulting in diminished protection. Although we have the same number of immune cells, they do not respond as quickly or effectively against potential enemies. Some of these changes may be programmed events that are part of the normal aging process, but I believe—and there are numerous studies to back me up—that poor diet and lifestyle accelerates the decline in immune function. Abusing your body by smoking, drinking heavily, living under a great deal of stress, not exercising, or eating poorly leaves you with an immune system that acts like it is old, no matter what its age. The good news is that even if you are older, you can rejuvenate your immune system by taking the right immunotics and maintaining a healthy lifestyle.

In many cases, the decline in immune function may be a result of decades of micronutrient starvation. To make matters worse, many older people do not eat well or skip meals altogether. The importance of diet is underscored by a recent Canadian study in which researchers gave a flu vaccine to 30 older people with poor eating habits. In addition to the flu shot, half the group was then given a nutritious diet while the others continued to eat a less nutritious diet. Four weeks later, the researchers found that those patients who ate a better diet had significantly more antibodies to flu virus than those who did not eat as well, an indication of improved immune function. If just four weeks of good nutrition can have such a profound effect on immune function, just think what years or decades of good nutrition and immunotics supplements can do!

Immunosenescence is not inevitable as long as you take

the necessary steps to prevent or reverse it. The Immunotics program is designed to keep your immune system running well into your senior years. It can even rejuvenate an older, damaged immune system; but the earlier you get started, the better.

## Immunonaive: The Young Immune System

During the first three months of life, the immune system is immature, leaving the newborn vulnerable to illness. At the first sign of trouble, therefore, many doctors automatically prescribe antibiotics for infants to prevent a small problem from becoming a more serious one. While well-intentioned, this may not always be the wisest thing to do. During this period, the immune system is learning some important lessons, and bombarding a baby with antibiotics may interfere with its development. However, I do want to stress that in some cases, antibiotics may be absolutely necessary. If you have any doubt as to the health of your newborn, consult your physician.

Obviously, since infants are defenseless, their mothers must help them avoid getting sick during this vulnerable time. As noted earlier, breast-feeding is a wonderful way for a mother to pass important immune factors onto her baby. It is particularly important for the newborn to get colostrum, special premilk produced during the first 48 hours by the mother.

Second, the parents of a newborn should take pains to protect their own health and the health of other children so they don't inadvertently pass infection on to their immunonaive infant. When you bring a newborn into the house, everyone must take care not to get sick. Strictly adhere to common-sense precautions, such as routine hand-washing, keeping sick people away from the infant, and keeping the infant away from crowds.

The new mother should keep her own immune system in tip-top form. She needs to make sure that she doesn't get sick and pass it on to her child. It is especially important for her to practice an immune-enhancing lifestyle. That means avoiding activities that dampen immune function (such as smoking and high alcohol consumption), eating the right foods to avoid micronutrient deficiencies, and getting enough sleep. I also advise nursing mothers to avoid eating foods that are filled with pesticides and other toxins. These can be passed through breast milk to infants and hamper their immune function. If ever there was a time to eat organic food, this is it. (See the discussion of toxic overload that follows the next section.)

## Immunodeficiency Disorders

Immunodeficiency disorders consist of a wide range of health problems—some congenital, some acquired—that interfere with the ability of the immune system to work effectively. There are about 70 hereditary immunodeficiency disorders that usually appear at birth and are characterized by a malfunction in some aspect of the immune system. Whatever the cause—not enough white blood cells or some other missing component—the net result is a lifelong increase in vulnerability to disease. An obvious sign of an immunodeficiency disorder is serious, chronic infection that does not respond to normal treatment. Generally, people with this problem get sick faster, more severely, and more often than normal and have an extremely difficult time shaking off an infection. Depending on the degree of impairment, immunodeficiency disorders can be debilitating or even fatal. Undoubtedly many of you have heard of the so-called bubble children, whose immune systems are so weak that they must live in a germ-free, hermetically sealed environment. That, thank goodness, is rare. In less serious forms of immunodeficiency, children can maintain a somewhat normal life, but they must take great precautions not to get sick.

The vast majority of immunodeficiency disorders strike later in life and are usually triggered by a disease such as diabetes, cancer, severe infections (such as measles), Down's syndrome, or kidney failure. Of course, the most notorious immunodeficiency disease is acquired immune deficiency syndrome (AIDS). Sometimes it is not the disease but its treatment that suppresses the immune response. The underlying disease may be under control, but the patient may succumb to an unrelated infection caused by the treatment. Organ transplantation and the potent immunosuppressive drugs needed to prevent organ rejection also trigger a temporary kind of immunodeficiency disorder. Even seemingly unrelated physical problems, such as trauma from a severe injury or surgery, can also cause immunodeficiency. With so much energy being channeled into healing that wound, the body simply doesn't have the resources to mount a serious immune defense against infection. If you are recovering from a wound or surgery in a germ-laden environment such as a hospital, you and your physician need to ensure that you stay as free from infection as possible.

If you have been diagnosed with an immunodeficiency

disorder or are undergoing medical treatment that may dampen immune function, you must protect your health. In this case, prevention really is the best medicine. Be especially vigilant about maintaining good nutrition, getting enough rest, avoiding harmful drugs and toxins, and steering clear of sick people. Check with your physician about getting appropriate vaccinations for flu or pneumonia. Use the Immunotics program to help you maintain as strong an immune system as possible.

## Toxic Overload

Excessive exposure to toxic substances can have a harmful effect on immune function. Our bodies have an elaborate mechanism to purify potentially poisonous chemicals, which is key to our survival. While it may seem like a no-brainer to avoid toxins—no health-conscious person will knowingly move near a toxic waste dump—it's not that simple. Our environment contains numerous toxins. With every breath we take, with every meal we eat, and with every beverage we drink, we take in thousands of potential poisons. Insecticides in food and water, cleaning fluids used at home and at work, chemicals commonly used on the job, and even prescription drugs can be dangerous substances. Even our bodies conspire against us. Many of the substances produced as part of normal metabolism are highly toxic. We are constantly challenging our bodies with more and more new toxins: about a thousand new chemicals each year! According to the U. S. Environmental Protection Agency, in 1994 more than 2 .2 *billion* pounds of toxic chemicals were released into the environment in the United States.

Many of us add to this toxic burden by knowingly ingesting poisons. Cigarettes, excess alcohol, and illicit drugs introduce a toxic cocktail of chemicals into our bodies. The burden of detoxification falls to the liver. The liver produces large amounts of the antioxidant glutathione, an essential part of the detoxification process. When glutathione encounters toxic compounds, it attaches to them and triggers a chemical reaction that flushes the toxins through the kidneys. When we are in toxic overload, however, our livers cannot keep up the pace.

Inadequately purified toxins can wreak havoc on every system of the body, including the immune system. Many toxins promote the formation of free radicals, thus depleting our stores of antioxidants. When antioxidants are depleted by toxic overload, there are not enough left to work with the immune system when we need them. Excessive toxins also shift the immune system into overdrive, thereby causing inflammation that can destroy healthy tissues.

Toxins can directly weaken immune cells as well. Numerous studies show that immune cells exposed to pollutants commonly found in the environment lose some of their zip. In particular, there is a decline in NK cell activity, making us more vulnerable to a host of infections and cancer. In high enough doses, toxins poison bone marrow, the heart of the immune system itself.

We cannot eliminate all toxins from our lives—that is neither practical or desirable. Few of us want to give up our cars or the conveniences of modern living, and we don't need to. But it is wise to reduce our exposure to unnecessary toxins. Whenever possible, I buy organic produce that has not been sprayed with insecticides. If you can't buy organic produce, rinse your fruits and vegetables thoroughly to remove pesticide residue, peeling them when necessary. Many of us are exposed to pesticides from the chemicals that we or our neighbors use on home lawns and gardens. If possible, switch to natural gardening methods. Ask your neighbors to notify you when they are going to be using pesticides—you may want to stay indoors or be away on those days. Try to reduce exposure to potentially harmful chemicals in your home or workplace. Fortunately, there are many cleansers, paper goods, and other products on the market that are made with less toxic materials. These products not only are good for the outside environment but are better for your internal one as well. Finally, avoid smoking, drinking excessive amounts of alcohol, and consuming processed foods laden with unnecessary chemicals.

## Living or Working in an Infection-Prone Environment

Some people, because of where they live or work, are continually overtaxing their immune systems. Not surprisingly, these people frequently show up in my office suffering from virus after virus, cold after cold. If you find yourself in any of the following categories, try to keep your immune system in peak condition.

### Hospital Workers and Patients

When it comes to catching an infection, one of the most dangerous places to be these days is a hospital. Day in and day out, hospital workers interact with countless numbers of sick people, many with infectious illnesses. Obviously, hospital workers who provide hands-on care for patients are at the greatest risk, but so are patients—even more so because of whatever problem landed them in the hospital in the first place! Two million infections are contracted in hospitals each year. This accounts for up to 80,000 deaths. Infectious organisms don't stay confined to the patient's room; they can be transmitted through the air or picked up on a doorknob or a magazine in the waiting room, and they gather on clothing, blankets, and medical equipment. If you work in a hospital, or know that you are going to be a patient, you must take every step you can to keep your immune system healthy.

## Exposure to Small Children

There is a reason why parents of preschool children and daycare workers are frequently ill. As their immune systems mature, small children are especially vulnerable to colds, flus, and viruses. While this is good for their immune systems—it teaches valuable lessons—it is hard on the rest of us. Because of poor hygiene (kids are not particularly good about hand washing) and close exposure to others, kids' colds and other ailments spread like wildfire to their friends, teachers, and family members. Some of this is unavoidable: When your child has a fever of 102 degrees, you need to give him a hug and kiss regardless of the consequences. (That's doctor's orders!) Try to teach kids the basics of good hygiene so that they reduce the risk of passing their illnesses on to others.

## The Closed Environment

You're at work at your cubicle in a modern office building. There are no windows in sight. The person in the next cubicle has a terrible cold and a hacking cough. Within a day or two, you and dozens of your coworkers also have the "office cold."

As a result of energy conservation measures taken in the 1970s and 1980s, many modern office buildings are closed environments: They do not have windows that can be opened to the outside. Air is recirculated through heating and ventilation systems, depositing your neighbor's virus in your lungs. Although closed buildings may reduce energy bills, they only enhance your risk of getting sick.

If you travel on an airplane, the air quality can be even worse. As part of cost-cutting measures, many airlines have reduced the amount of fresh air they pump into the cabins; instead they recycle old air. The germs sneezed out by a passenger in first class can quickly find their way back to row 32! The only antidote to the closed environment is fresh air. Back in Hippocrates' day, physicians urged everyone to get ample amounts of fresh air daily. That's good advice. If you work in a closed building, take a walk during the day to fill your lungs with fresh air. There are also steps you can take to clean up your work environment, which I explain in chapter 9. If you are a frequent flier (with the accompanying frequent respiratory problems) follow the Immunotics program for people in high-risk work or family situations.

## Overexposure to Antibiotics

I explained earlier how overexposure to antibiotics has hurt society by creating antibiotic-resistant organisms. In addition, when you overuse and abuse antibiotics you harm yourself. Several studies have documented that overuse of antibiotics can dampen immune function, leaving you more vulnerable than ever to illness. For example, long-term use of sulfa drugs (a type of antibiotic) causes a decline in white blood-cell count, which weakens the immune system. Other studies have documented that antibiotics can reduce levels of cytokines, the hormonal messengers in the immune system that are instrumental in fighting disease. Perversely, the more you use antibiotics, the more you need them. While they help to fight one infection, they weaken your body's ability to fight the next one.

Antibiotics also cause harm by killing the good bacteria in the gut. Without enough good bacteria in your intestinal tract, your immune system has to work harder to maintain the proper balance of microorganisms and fight off bacteria, fungi, and parasites. You can correct some, but not all, of the negative effects of antibiotics by taking the probiotic supplements I describe in chapter 4.

I worry about children who have been given too many antibiotics, especially for problems like ear infections that generally do not warrant antibiotic use. Earlier I noted that a child's immune system must learn how to live in a world filled with threatening organisms. With each viral and bacterial infection, it gleans an important lesson on survival. By giving a child an antibiotic for every problem, we prevent the immune system from doing its job and learning these important lessons. It's as foolish as keeping your child out of school.

## Sleep Deprivation

Have you ever noticed that when you don't get enough sleep and feel run-down, you are a magnet for every bug that comes your way? It's not just your imagination—sleep deprivation can have a powerfully detrimental effect on your immune system.

Sleep deprivation is an extremely common problem in

the United States, so common in fact that it is one of the primary complaints I hear from my patients. In fact, about 100 million Americans have sleep problems at one time or another. While anxiety, depression, side effects from medication, and hormonal changes due to aging can all contribute to sleep problems, they are not entirely responsible for the epidemic of sleep deprivation in the United States. In many—if not most—cases, people are simply so busy that they don't set aside enough time to sleep.

I fault our society's "push yourself until you drop" philosophy. I mentioned earlier how when patients get sick, they expect an instant cure, not a few days in bed. If we don't give ourselves time to rest when we are sick, we certainly won't do so when we are well. We expect ourselves (and others) to GO GO GO. We never give our bodies enough downtime. In our society, sleep has become a luxury; to some, it's even a weakness! But it is very much a necessity of life.

While we sleep, our bodies are performing two essential tasks. The first and most obvious role of sleep is to give our bodies a chance to rest and refuel. During sleep, our heart rate and blood pressure drop, and our metabolism (the process by which our bodies use energy) slows down. Because it takes less steam to run our bodies during sleep, our cells can concentrate on the second vital task: repairing and creating new cells in every system of the body, including the immune system.

What happens to the immune system when we are deprived of sleep? A psychiatrist at San Diego Veterans Affairs Medical Center monitored 23 healthy men ages 22 to 61 for four nights at a sleep laboratory. For the first two nights, they were allowed to sleep normally, but on the third night, they were denied sleep between 3 A.M. and 7 A.M. After the sleep-less night, the men showed dramatic changes in immune function, notably a decline in natural killer cell activity. This means that they were more vulnerable to infection. However, when the men were allowed to sleep normally the following night, their immune systems bounced back to normal.

Clearly, adequate sleep is important for a strong immune system. If you don't sleep enough, examine your lifestyle to determine if you are sabotaging your good night's sleep in some way. For example, caffeinated or alcoholic beverages too close to bedtime can disrupt sleep patterns. So can vigorous exercise. You may be too stressed out by the end of the day to get a good night's rest. The important thing is to understand why sleep is important and do everything you can to make sure you get enough of it. It's your body's basic currency, and you never want to run short of cash, right?

## Excessive Stress

When you are under a great deal of stress for an extended period of time, you put your immune system at risk. There is compelling scientific evidence that chronic stress causes a measurable decline in the immune system's ability to fight disease.

Of course, everybody experiences stressful situations every day. We must put up with momentary traffic jams, demanding bosses, family squabbles, and difficult deadlines. And to top it off, we always feel pressed for time. These normal stressors, however, are usually transient and do not exact a steep toll on us physically or emotionally. Others can be more profound and long-lasting. They hit us longer and harder than the usual stresses of daily living. The loss of a job, the death of a spouse or child, a severe disappointment, the breakup of a marriage—these are all examples of situations that can trigger a vigorous stress response in the body.

When we encounter a stressful situation—whether it is an angry boss or an emotional trauma—our brains send our adrenal glands a signal to start pumping out stress hormones: the so-called fight-or-flight response. Stress hormones trigger a chain of reactions that prepare our bodies for an emergency. Our blood pressure rises, our hearts pump faster, our pupils dilate, and we are ready for action. Within a short time, our bodies return to normal, and we are none the worse for the experience. However, under constant stress, the continual bombardment of stress hormones can have a harmful effect on many different body systems, especially the immune system. Studies have shown that after periods of extreme stress, our T-cells do not work efficiently. For example, people who have recently lost a spouse typically show a marked drop in immune function. People who are depressed often have depressed NK cell activity. Most doctors will confirm that patients experiencing shock, sadness, or grief are very vulnerable to illness. In my practice, I have noticed that the patients who fare the worst are the ones who are so overwhelmed that they feel out of control of their lives. Understanding and controlling stress is so important to immune health that I devote a good deal of my practice counseling patients on stress management. For more information, see chapter 9.

## Strenuous Physical Exercise

While moderate exercise is good for you and can even enhance immune health, too much exercise can overtax your immune system. It is a well-known fact that marathon runners are particularly vulnerable to respiratory infections during their intense training period and immediately following the marathon. Why? When you are engaged in intense physical activity—whether it is running, kickboxing, or pumping iron—you burn more oxygen, which in turn produces more free radicals. As noted earlier, excessive amounts of free radicals deplete antioxidants and *dampen* immune response. If you do any form of vigorous exercise, be sure to replenish the lost antioxidants through food and supplements.

Competitive activities like marathon running can also be very stressful, especially if you are intent on winning or placing in the top percentile. Any kind of stress—physical or emotional—increases the level of stress hormones, which in turn can inhibit immune response. If you have your heart set on marathon running or engaging in other equally strenuous activities, be sure that your immune system is well fortified by following the program listed in chapter 6.

## Too Much Sun

I have noticed that many of my patients who vacation in tropical paradises often return from their trips with the same complaint: They say that within a day of starting their vacations, they got sick. Typically, they are stuck in bed with a very nasty cold—and a very nasty disposition! When I ask these patients how they spent their time before they got sick, they usually reply that they were basking in the sun for hours. This is a bad idea, and not just for the obvious reasons. We all know that the sun can cause severe damage to skin, causing premature aging and even skin cancer. What is less well known is that the intense exposure to the sun can dampen immune function! Here's why. First, ultraviolet (UV) radiation from the sun causes the formation of free radicals, depleting the body of important antioxidants. Second, UV radiation may also raise levels of stress hormones, which also dampen immune function, as just mentioned. The bottom line is, be careful about too much exposure to the sun. And if you're planning a tropical vacation, be sure to follow the Immunotics program for travelers on pages 157 to 158.

Enough about all the risk factors and behaviors we should all avoid. Now, it's time to discuss solutions. The next chapter introduces you to a powerful new tool in getting healthy—and staying healthy.

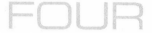

# The Immunotics Pharmacy

**H**ere we are at the core of the book: the Immunotics pharmacy. This is the medicine cabinet of the book, where you can find all you need to know about each of the immunotics. You may be familiar with some of the better known ones, like garlic and cranberry, but I think you'll be surprised by the solid scientific and clinical evidence confirming the medicinal properties of these traditional favorites. Other immunotics, such as colostrum and astragalus, may be completely new to you. This chapter tells when, how, and who should use all these supplements.

Immunotics serve two purposes: Either they can boost your immune system on a preventive, ongoing basis or they can be treatments for common ailments if you do get sick. Just like you don't take the same antibiotic for every infection, you should not use the same immunotic for every ailment or condition. As you'll read, some immunotics are quite potent. Like any other strong medicine, you want to save them for when they are really needed. Price and availability is also a factor. Some immunotics are relatively expensive or more difficult to obtain; therefore, I recommend them only when nothing else will work as well. You will notice that with many immunotics, I give a range of doses rather than a specific dose. Doses vary depending on how the immunotic is being used. At lower doses, many immunotics are excellent overall immune enhancers, but in higher doses, the same immunotics are effective treatments for acute problems. I note the maintenance dose and the treatment dose. Second, not everyone responds the same way to drugs or supplements. Some people are highly sensitive to even low doses, while others require much higher doses to get the same effect. Figuring out the right dose for you is a trial-and-error process called titration. Chapters 6 and 7 tell you how to use the immunotics discussed here to maintain your health and conquer specific problems.

Supplements should be taken with food unless otherwise specified. (For more information on how to take supplements, see chapter 6.)

This chapter also reviews the science behind Immunotics. There are thousands of scientific studies, but for obvious reasons I highlight only the most important. For a more complete list of references, turn to the bibliography at the end of the book.

In most cases, I recommend using any of the high-quality

products available for each immunotic. In some special cases, I recommend a specific product brand or brands. An asterisk after the supplement name tells you that I have a special brand recommendation. In the interest of full disclosure, I do have to note that I have designed my own brand of immunotics. However, I am presenting the supplement regimens in generic terms with appropriate doses so you can obtain them from whatever source you find most convenient and economical. The recommended products are listed in the resources section at the end of the book.

### Aloe Vera*

**Rx:**  The herbal immunotic for GI problems.

**The Right Amount:**  Range: ½ to 2 teaspoons of freeze-dried aloe daily. Aloe vera is available in juice or gel. The gel is more expensive. I recommend a daily aloe gel supplement to people who have *chronic* gut problems and aloe juice for those with *acute* problems. Lower chronic dose: mix ½ teaspoon of freeze-dried aloe powder with a small amount of water once or twice daily and take before meals. Higher chronic dose: mix ½ teaspoon of freeze-dried aloe leaf powder daily with a small amount of water up to 4 times daily, before meals. For acute problems: drink 2 ounces of juice every 2 hours for up to 12 hours.

For nearly four thousand years, the aloe vera plant (*Aloe barbadenis*) has been valued for its medicinal purposes, and for good reason. I've found it invaluable in treating both chronic and acute gut problems, especially in the freeze-

dried form (listed in the resources section). It not only promotes healing of the gut but also enhances immune function
throughout the gastrointestinal tract. You probably know of
aloe already and, if you're anything like me, have sung its
praises when you're sunburned! The leaf of the aloe plant
contains the special gel or natural emollient that is used in
many skin care products. When used topically, aloe gel is a
mild antiseptic and anti-inflammatory that promotes the
healing of wounds and burns. It can also soothe your insides,
relieving the symptoms of peptic ulcers and cooling off an
angry gut. The lining of our GI tract and cavity resembles the
skin, and when our gut is injured, it uses the same healing
mechanisms as skin. This is not just theory. I have prescribed
freeze-dried aloe gel to hundreds of patients with GI problems, with excellent results.

As you already know, the gut is a major component of the
immune system, and anything that attacks the gut hurts our
ability to keep all disease at bay. In fact, the gut contains
more immune cells than any other part of the body. Maintaining gut health is essential for a strong immune system,
and vice versa. Aloe gel can help on this front as well. Specifically, aloe gel boosts the activity of macrophages in the gut—
immune cells that gobble up bad bacteria, viruses, and other
nasty pathogens.

Let me clear up one point of confusion about aloe. Some
physicians and herbal healers warn against taking aloe inter-
nally. They are talking about aloe *rind,* not aloe pulp. The
rind of the aloe contains aloin and emodin, two powerful
cathartics that some natural healers use as a laxative. In fact,
I don't even recommend aloe rind as a laxative. It can be ter-
ribly harsh and cause severe cramping. Aloe pulp, however,

contains no aloin and has no laxative properties. It is perfectly safe.

Aloe is available in juice or gel. The juice is gel that has
been reconstituted with water, preservatives, and flavorings.
It is not as potent as the gel but is fine for occasional GI problems like stomach flu. For chronic problems, however, the
gel is better.

### Alkylglycerol (Shark Liver Oil) *

**Rx:** Strengthens an aging or weak immune system;
provides postoperative and cancer protection; an essential immunotic for people working or living in a
high-risk environment.

**The Right Amount:** Range: 750–1500 mg daily. Lower
dose: take 1 (250 mg) capsule 3 times daily. Higher
dose: take 1 (500 mg) capsule 3 times daily.

Alkylglycerol—as bone marrow—has been used as a component of folk medicine for hundreds of years. Today, alkylglycerol shows great promise as an adjuvant therapy to
conventional cancer treatment, but it is also a superb immunotic for anyone who needs an extra boost. I prescribe
alkylglycerol for patients who are undergoing chemotherapy
or radiation. I also recommend it for anyone who lives or
works in a high-risk environment, such as parents of small
children, teachers, and hospital workers. If you're having a
bad winter—if you're constantly battling cold after cold and
flu after flu—alkylglycerol could help turn things around.

Shark liver oil has a particularly interesting history that re-
minds us that we should not dismiss folk remedies as unsci-

entific nonsense. Sometimes it just takes a few hundred years for science to catch up! For centuries, sailors and fishermen told tales of the amazing healing abilities of sharks. Injured sharks, they said, mended practically overnight. Just another fish story, right? In fact, fishermen have long used shark liver oil as a folk remedy to treat skin wounds, and in 1922, Japanese scientists isolated alkylglycerols—lipidlike compounds—from shark liver oil, which became the subject of intense scientific research. Sharks were not the only animals that produced alkylglycerols. The same compound was found in human breast milk (which also has immune-boosting properties) and in the bone marrow of cows. Nevertheless, no one understood what it did.

In 1952, Swedish physician Astrid Brohult was seeking a treatment for children with leukemia to mitigate the serious side effects of chemotherapy. As you already know, chemotherapy inhibits the production of immune cells within the bone marrow, resulting in an increased risk of infection. Too often, cancer patients fall victim to sepsis, a blood infection that sends them back to the hospital. Low white-blood-cell count is one of the most significant complications from chemotherapy. Dr. Brohult knew that calves, like humans, produce white blood cells in their marrow. She decided to feed her young charges hefty portions of calf marrow to boost their white-blood-cell count. (Interestingly, bone marrow is a longtime folk remedy for anemia and other blood diseases.) Dr. Brohult noticed a marked improvement in her patients. She wanted to conduct further studies on bone marrow. One problem arose. Have you ever tried to feed a kid bone marrow . . . in large quantities? Dr. Brohult and her husband, a chemist, sought a way to make bone marrow palatable to children—they even mixed it with chocolate! However, in refining it, they discovered that alkylglycerol was the active ingredient in marrow: alkylglycerol, the same lipidlike substance found in the liver of the Greenland shark. (While alkylglycerol is present in all sharks, cold-water sharks have the highest concentration.) There were major benefits to using shark liver oil instead of bone marrow. Shark liver oil not only was a much more potent source of alkylglycerol than bone marrow but contained other beneficial compounds, including squalene, also being studied as a potential cancer fighter.

Alkylglycerol upgrades immune function in several ways. It stimulates the formation of helper T-cells, boosts macrophage production, and heightens NK cell activity. Studies conducted by Dr. Brohult and others showed that shark liver oil given prior to, during, and after radiation therapy can protect healthy tissue from damage while significantly reducing side effects. One major study suggests that radiation combined with shark liver oil improves the chances of survival. Two thousand–plus women with cervical cancer were divided into two groups. One was given standard radiation therapy alone, and the other was given radiation plus shark liver oil supplements during the treatment. After five years, the survival rate for the radiation-alone group was 50 percent, but the survival rate for the radiation-plus-shark-liver-oil group was 65 percent, a notable increase.

Promising animal studies have shown that shark liver oil can reduce metastasis (the spread of cancer cells beyond the original site) in animals with mammary cancers. This suggests that it may be useful in the prevention of a recurrence.

Shark liver oil has even been used topically to treat skin cancer.

I have prescribed alkylglycerol to many patients undergoing cancer treatment, with excellent results. In fact, many patients grinningly report that their oncologists are amazed at how strong their immune function is despite their cancer treatment. Alkylglycerol is very safe and utterly nontoxic. Frankly, I don't know why all oncologists don't use it routinely.

---

### Antioxidants

**Rx:** A building block of a healthy immune system. Everyone should take a daily antioxidant supplement, but it is especially important for people over 50 and endurance athletes.

**The Right Amount:** As part of the Basic Immunotics Program, I prescribe an antioxidant complex containing at least five key antioxidants:

| | |
|---|---|
| *Vitamin E:* | take 400 international units (IUs) daily (1 IU is equal to 1 mg). |
| *Vitamin C:* | take between 1000 and 2000 mg daily. |
| *Zinc chelate:* | take between 25 and 50 mg daily. |
| *Selenomethionine:* | take between 100 and 200 mcg daily. |
| *Mixed carotenoids:* | take 15,000–30,000 mg daily. |

People with specific risk factors will need to take additional antioxidants (see chapter 6).

Antioxidants are a family of vitamins, minerals, and other nutrients that are vital for a robust immune system. Antioxidants are crucial to numerous body processes. Without antioxidants, we would not be able to wage a strong immune response. I recommend that everyone—men, women, and children—take an antioxidant supplement daily. In some cases, depending on specific risk factors, I may prescribe higher doses of certain antioxidants or additional antioxidants.

Antioxidants play a pivotal role in the immune system. They boost immune function, enabling immune cells to fight harder. At the same time, they protect us against free radicals, unstable molecules that are a normal byproduct of energy production in the body.

The human body requires ample amounts of energy for growth and other body activities, from breathing to the beating of our hearts. Oxygen is the fuel that turns on energy production. Yet the burning of oxygen can create free radicals, and they can damage cell structure and lead to chronic disease. Think of free radicals as small sparks in a forest—extinguished early on, they pose no threat. Left to spread, they can cause a catastrophe.

Free radicals are not all bad—in fact, they are one of the body's primary weapons against viruses, bacteria, and other invaders. When we are sick, we pump out more free radicals in the fight against dangerous pathogens. This is good, up to a point. Too many free radicals, however, can cause chronic inflammation that will damage healthy cells, including immune cells. Oxidative stress is a condition that occurs when the body has too many free radicals and too few antioxidants. The cure to oxidative stress is more antioxidants to neutralize excess free radicals. You can maintain the right balance between antioxidants and free radicals through proper diet and by taking the right supplements.

Important antioxidants for immune health include vitamins C, E, glutathione, coenzyme Q-10, and lipoic acid, as well as phytochemicals such as carotenoids and bioflavonoids. (Bioflavonoids are effective immune enhancers in their own right but also greatly boost the power of vitamin C. See the special section on bioflavonoids later in this chapter.)

*Vitamin C* Thanks to the work of the late Linus Pauling, you have undoubtedly heard that vitamin C can help you recover faster from the common cold and may even help protect against cancer. What you may not know is that vitamin C performs its magic via the immune system. The concentration of vitamin C in immune cells is 20 to 100 times higher than in the rest of the blood. It is there for a reason. As shown by several studies, vitamin C boosts the activity of NK cells. It works fast, too. People who take vitamin C supplements see a measurable increase in NK activity within 24 hours. The Recommended Dietary Allowance (RDA) set for vitamin C by the National Academy of Sciences is 60 mg a day, but the RDAs are not about achieving optimal health. They are designed only to prevent outright deficiency. In reality, people need about 500 mg of vitamin C daily to maintain good immune health. Sadly, about 25 percent of the U. S. population does not consume even the low RDA of 60 mg of vitamin C daily.

*Vitamin E* Also known as tocopherol, vitamin E is not produced by the body and must be obtained through diet or supplements. Nutritionally, vitamin E is found in raw vegetable oils, nuts, and nut butters. Since we eat these high-caloric, high-fat foods in limited quantities, supplementation is essential. The RDA for vitamin E is 30 IU daily, but studies show at least 200 IU is needed for optimal immune function. Vitamin E is especially critical for older people experiencing the slowdown in immune function. In a recent study conducted at the U. S. Department of Agriculture's Human Nutrition Center at Tufts University, 88 people ages 65 and over were given either a placebo or 60, 200, or 800 IUs of vitamin E daily for four months. At the end of the four-month period, researchers reported an increase in T-cell and B-cell activity among the vitamin E takers. Moreover, those who took vitamin E showed a more vigorous immune response to the tetanus and hepatitis B vaccines, a sign of improved antibody production. As people age, their ability to produce antibodies is diminished. The people who took vitamin E noticed its effects as well, showing a 30 percent decrease in self-reported infections compared with the non–vitamin E takers.

*Lipoic acid* Instrumental in the production of energy by the cells of the body, lipoic acid is the ultimate team player. It greatly enhances the effect of other antioxidants, including vitamins C and E while elevating the levels of another important antioxidant, glutathione.

*Glutathione* This antioxidant is produced by the body from other compounds. Its many roles include the detoxification of drugs and pollutants and the maintenance of healthy liver function. The importance of glutathione is underscored by the fact that there is a direct correlation between health, longevity, and glutathione levels. Low levels of glutathione are a harbinger of illness and premature death. Adequate glutathione levels are essential for T-cell function, but chronic illness saps the body of glutathione. Glutathione is produced in the cells from three amino acids: cysteine, glutamic acid, and glycine. However, glutathione is not easy to supplement: the molecule is too big to pass readily from the digestive system into the cells. Consequently, very large doses are needed to absorb significant levels. However, it is possible to boost glutathione levels indirectly by eating the right foods—primarily fresh fruits such as oranges and watermelon, and vegetables such as broccoli, spinach, and tomatoes—and taking other antioxidants, such as vitamin C, lipoic acid, and the immunotic NAC.

*CoQ-10* Produced by every cell in the body, this antioxidant is found in small amounts in many different foods but primarily in organ meats. While CoQ-10 is important for immune health, it is critical for the production of energy in the body. More important, CoQ-10 works in synergy with vitamin E, boosting the effectiveness of each. CoQ-10 is good for everyone, but I recommend it especially for people over age 50 (since blood levels decline with age) and for athletes who, because of their higher energy needs, are often in oxidative stress.

*Carotenoids* Carotenoids are natural pigments found in both plants and animals. Fruits and vegetables rich in carotenoids are known for their bright colors, ranging from brilliant yellow, red, and orange to purple and dark green. There are about 60 carotenoids found in nature, including beta carotene, alpha carotene, lycopene, lutein, cryptoxanthin, and xeaxanthin. Numerous studies confirm that people who eat foods rich in carotenoids are less likely to get cancer or heart disease than those who don't. Carotenoids not only are antioxidants but are natural immune boosters that increase NK cell activity.

*Zinc* 30 percent of all people over 50 do not get enough zinc from their diet. Studies show, at any age, that people with the greatest zinc deficiencies have the poorest response to germs. Zinc supplements can boost blood levels of a chemical that is essential for the production of mature T-cells. Zinc can also help reduce the symptoms and the duration of the common cold, according to a study conducted at Dartmouth College. In fact, many of you already probably suck on a zinc lozenge at the first sign of a cold. Good thinking. It may help you kick the cold faster.

*Selenium* Glutathione is valuable in the body only when it is made chemically available, and that is where selenium comes in. Found in foods such as onion, garlic, and broccoli, this mineral is critical for the production of an enzyme that helps the body utilize glutathione efficiently. As a side benefit, selenium can also enhance the effectiveness of vitamin E. Low blood levels of selenium have been linked to an increased risk of cancer and a sluggish immune system. The modest RDA for selenium is 55 mcg for women and 75 mcg for men, yet most Americans do not even consume this amount in their daily diet. To make up for this deficiency, I recommend a form of selenium called selenomethionine, which is well absorbed by the body.

Some minerals are also important antioxidants. In particular, zinc and selenium, though essential for immune function, are frequently missing from our diets.

Don't worry, you're not going to have to go out and buy a

half a dozen different antioxidants. There are several antioxidant combination formulas on the market that include the antioxidants that are important for immune health. Antioxidants come in powders, tablets, pills, and even chewable tablets for children.

### Astragalus*

**Rx:**  A broad spectrum immunotic for people who are run-down and need an overall immune boost. Also an excellent adjuvant therapy to chemotherapy. I especially recommend astragalus to children who are having a bad winter and need to build their resistance!

**The Right Amount:**  Range: 1000–2000 mg daily or 1–4 dropperfuls of tincture. Lower dose: take 2 (500 mg) capsules daily or 2 dropperfuls of tincture. Higher dose: take 4 (500 mg) capsules daily or 4 dropperfuls of tincture.

Astragalus, known by the botanical name *astragalus membranaceus*, is an herb that has been used in traditional Chinese medicine for thousands of years to support the wei ch'i, or "defensive energy," of the body. While it is an excellent general tonic to support immune function and prevent illness, it can also be beneficial for acute infection, especially colds and flu.

The active ingredient in astragalus resembles the chemical structure of two other immunotics, echinacea and larch. Like those American herbs, astragalus enhances the activity of macrophages and boosts the production of superoxide ions and hydrogen peroxide, oxygen radicals that continue attacking the bad guys. To further support immune function, astragalus also ups both NK cell and T-cell activity.

Cancer devastates the immune system. In addition to the immunosuppressive effects of conventional therapies, the cancerous tumors themselves produce substances that suppress macrophage function, inhibiting the body's ability to fight the cancer as well as other illnesses. Cancer leaves you in a weakened, defenseless state, but astragalus may help cancer patients maintain normal immune function. According to a study conducted by researchers at Loma Linda University in Loma Linda, California, published in the *Journal of Urology,* an extract derived from astragalus (combined with another Chinese herb, ligustrum) can reverse the suppression of macrophage activity by bladder tumors in mice. The researchers noted: "This lends further support to the concept that aqueous extracts of traditional Chinese herbs may indeed act as biological response modifiers due to the presence of one or more extremely potent, naturally occurring immune stimulants."

Researchers at the University of Texas Medical Center in Houston have also seen benefits. They found that astragalus extract helps to normalize the immune systems of cancer patients with impaired immunity due to chemotherapy.

I recommend astragalus to my patients who are getting sick more than usual and are feeling run-down. In particular, I prescribe astragalus to children who are having a bad winter, suffering with chronic colds, flus, and ear infections. Along with other immunotics, over time it seems to give them the added boost they need to get well and stay well.

You may find it surprising that the same immunotic used for cancer is also useful for something as benign as the com-

mon cold. In reality, what is good for restoring immune function in cancer patients is also good for helping the body fight
against *all* infection. These immunotics, though potent, do
you no harm. They can be strong enough to help tackle a
cancer and gentle enough to treat a child's sniffles.

---

### Berberine*

**Rx:** Nature's antibiotic, good for stomach bugs, colds,
flus, and other infections. For occasional use only.

**The Right Amount:** Range: 300–1200 mg daily of
berberine capsules or 1–4 dropperfuls of tincture (derived from plant extract). Lower dose: take 1 dropperful of tincture (300 mg) daily for up to 14 days. Higher
dose: take 4 dropperfuls of tincture (1200 mg) daily for
up to 14 days.

---

Berberine is a natural antibiotic found primarily in three
widely used traditional healing herbs: goldenseal (*Hydrastis
canadensis*), Oregon grape (*Berberis aquifolium*), and barberry
(*Berberis vulgaris*). Berberine's antibiotic activity targets bacteria—including those that commonly cause food poisoning—parasites, and fungi. I often recommend it to people
who are prone to traveler's diarrhea, in that berberine works
particularly well for acute bacterial diarrhea. Studies have
shown that berberine is effective against several common
bugs that wreak havoc on the GI tract, and *Shigella dysenteriae,*
the cause of shigellosis. Berberine does not appear to hurt
the normal flora found in the gut, nor does it promote the
development of antibiotic-resistant bugs. I often use it in
place of the antibiotic Cipro, which may beat the infections

but in the process also may harm beneficial intestinal flora. In addition, natural healers use berberine to treat yeast infections.

Berberine is not just a natural analogue of synthetic antibiotics. To the contrary, berberine has immune-enhancing, not immune-dampening, properties. It helps the immune system fight its own battles by boosting macrophage activity. At normally prescribed levels for short periods of time, berberine is nontoxic; however, at higher doses (well beyond what I prescribe) it can interfere with the metabolism of B vitamins. Berberine is often sold in combination capsules with other immunotics such as echinacea. In fact, I often recommend a combination berberine-echinacea formula for my patients. (Do not use berberine during pregnancy.)

## Bioflavonoids

**Rx:** Great antioxidants that fortify the body against infection, take the sting out of allergies, and soothe inflammation.

**The Right Amount:** The right amount depends on which bioflavonoid you use and why you are using it. Mixed citrus bioflavonoids: take up to 2500 mg daily. Quercetin: take up to 3000 mg daily. Proanthocyanidins: take between 150 and 300 mg daily.

Bioflavonoids are a group of more than four thousand different compounds found in plant pigments Remarkably, at least half of all bioflavonoids are also antioxidants, and several are proven immune boosters. About 50 bioflavonoids are present in common plant foods and beverages, such as

berries, citrus fruits, apples, onions, tea, and wine. If you eat
a diet rich in plant foods, you are already getting a substan-
tial dose of bioflavonoids. Nevertheless, it may not be
enough. Our bodies do not absorb these nutrients efficiently. Only about 10 percent of the bioflavonoids in food
are absorbed by the body. Depending on your health, your
immune system may need more than is available from food
to function at its optimal level. And if you're like the majority of Americans who don't eat the recommended five servings of fruits and vegetables daily, you may be seriously
deficient in these important micronutrients.

Supplemental bioflavonoids are available in two forms:
mixed citrus bioflavonoids and individual bioflavonoids.
Mixed citrus bioflavonoids, as the name implies, are a blend
of many different kinds of bioflavonoids into one prepara-
tion. You can also purchase individual bioflavonoids (such as
quercetin, grapeseed extract, pine bark extract, or proanthocyanidins) to meet specific challenges. Bioflavonoids are
so safe and nontoxic that I recommend mixed citrus bioflavonoids for everybody—children and adults—who needs
immune support. I reserve individual bioflavonoids for specific problems.

While bioflavonoid compounds have long been used in
traditional medicine, modern science did not discover them
until they were officially identified and isolated by Nobel
Laureate Albert Szent-Gyorgyi, who gained fame as the first
scientist to isolate vitamin C. Szent-Gyorgyi called bioflavonoids vitamin P and observed that these chemicals appeared to have an unexplained synergistic relationship with
vitamin C. Today we know that bioflavonoids enhance vita-

min C activity in the body. At times it is difficult to tell where the effect of one ends and the other begins.

Bioflavonoids are accessory nutrients; that is, they do not prevent any specific deficiency disease, but they have an important role in the body. In the 1960s, physicians prescribed bioflavonoids to treat problems such as gum disease and circulatory disorders, but after the USDA issued a report dismissing bioflavonoids as worthless in the 1970s, the medical community turned away from them.

We now know that these micronutrients may be worth their weight in gold. Numerous studies have documented that people who eat a diet rich in bioflavonoids enjoy a lower risk of developing cardiovascular disease and cancer.

When it comes to immune function, bioflavonoids perform wonders. They stimulate NK cell activity. They also increase the production of interleukin 2, a substance that promotes the activity of disease-fighting T-cells and lymphocytes. They help prevent the inevitable inflammation that occurs when the immune system goes into high gear. They do so many things that I wonder how we could have ignored them for so long!

Special problems need special solutions, and that is where individual bioflavonoids come in. While the mixed bioflavonoids are a superlative general-purpose booster, individual ones shine when you really need them. However, they are more expensive.

Mother Nature has designed an ingenious system to ensure the survival of mammalian babies (including humans) during the first few days of life when their immune systems are still highly underdeveloped. Not a high-tech antibiotic or

*Quercetin* Quercetin, which is found in abundance in the skins of apples and yellow and red onions is the bioflavonoid I recommend to my patients with hay fever or asthma. An allergic reaction occurs when the immune system overreacts to a normally harmless substance such as pollen. As you may remember from chapter 2, white blood cells produce the allergic antibody IgE, which stimulates an eruption of mast cells. Mast cells are the main storage sites for histamine, a chemical that is essential for digestion and the dilation of small blood vessels but that in excess can cause the usual unpleasant allergic symptoms such as teary eyes, swelling, and congestion. Quercetin helps to stabilize mast cells. In effect, it calms down those excitable cells, preventing an over-release of histamine. It is similar in action to the prescription drug cromolyn, marketed under the names Intal, Nasalcom, Crolom, and Gastrocrom. Quercetin also has strong antiviral activity, particularly against herpes, so I recommend it to people with serious viral infections. An added bonus: in numerous preliminary studies, quercetin has been shown to block the action of several known carcinogens. This is an immunotic to watch.

*Proanthocyanidins* Proanthocyanidins (PCOs) are a special variety of bioflavonoids found in the blue, purple, and green pigments of plants. Blueberries, cranberries, and grapes, for example, are terrific food sources of proanthocyanidins. It's well known that cranberries can help protect against bladder and urinary tract infections. Until recently, scientists believed that the acidic content of cranberries killed the bacteria causing the infection. However, why the acidity only targeted the bladder was never explained. We know now that the real credit goes to the PCOs, which prevent the bacteria from adhering to the bladder wall. (Blueberries offer the same protection!) There are several different supplement sources of PCOs on the market, including pine bark extract (and the brand Pycnogenol, a patented form) and grape seed extract. As far as I'm concerned, they are all excellent. PCOs do what other bioflavonoids do, only better—they are the Cadillac of bioflavonoids. They may cost more, but a small amount goes a long way. Since PCOs tend to be more expensive than mixed bioflavonoids, I recommend them for people who really need them: people with cancer or chronic immune weakness, people under severe oxidative stress, and people with autoimmune disorders. (In addition to being wonderful immune boosters, they are excellent for circulatory problems such as varicose veins.) Of course, if your budget allows, there's no reason why you can't take PCOs every day. You'll be healthier for the investment.

**Colostrum\***

**Rx:** Part of the Basic Immunotics Program for everyone. Colostrum works best for people with *chronic* conditions, such as yeast overgrowth, long-term respiratory
infections, and GI woes, but is also an excellent treatment for stomach flu. I highly recommend it for an aging immune system, for people living or working in a
high-risk environment, and after surgery.

**The Right Amount:** Range: 1440 to 4320 mg. (The brand
of colostrum I recommend comes in 480 mg tablets.)
Lower dose: take 3 (480 mg) capsules daily on an empty
stomach for general health. For higher dose: take 2–3
(480 mg) capsules *3* times daily (or a total of 9).

**Special Instructions:** Always take colostrum on an
empty stomach.

an exotic-sounding herb—it's plain old mother's milk. From
this unique creation of nature comes bovine *colostrum*—the
immunotic of choice for chronic, long-term problems. It's
essential when you need a general tuning up of the immune
system, and it is the first thing I reach for when I'm burning
the candle at both ends. Literally hundreds of my patients
swear by it. Taken daily as an overall immune enhancer—or
with other immunotics as a "shot in the arm" when you are
sick—colostrum works wonders. I have a few patients who
obtain theirs fresh off the farm (I live in Colorado, after all);
for the rest of us, a freeze-dried form is easily available in capsule or powder from natural food stores and pharmacies.

Mother's milk is best for newborns. Breast-fed infants
have a lower incidence of ear infections, colds, urinary tract

infections, and stomach bugs than formula-fed babies. We now know the reason why, as pediatricians say, breast milk is best. It contains, we've learned, a veritable pharmacy of immune-boosting proteins, and colostrum is the most potent part of breast milk.

The best immunotic of all is a naturally strong immune system. To establish that, I urge most women to breast-feed for at least the first six months. Colostrum, the milk produced during the first 48 hours after giving birth, is critical for the newborn's health, for now and for the child's whole lifetime.

Colostrum is "premilk"—a thin, yellowish fluid produced for only the first two days after giving birth by lactating hu-

*Lactoferrin* This protein binds to iron, which in excess can promote the growth of pathogenic bacteria. (That's why, when people have an infection, they are usually advised to stop taking iron supplements!) Interestingly, lactoferrin does not interfere with the absorption of iron by the body—in fact, it seems to facilitate it. However, it is the unbound iron, the iron not taken up by cells, that provides fuel for bacteria and promotes the formation of free radicals. Numerous studies document that lactoferrin also has natural antibiotic, antifungal, and possibly anticancer activity. Lactoferrin is not just for infants—it is found throughout the adult body as part of the immune system's defense against infection. According to a study published in *Cancer Research,* lactoferrin can inhibit both the growth of solid tumors and metastasis in mice. Refined lactoferrin is being tested as a potential cancer treatment and is used by some alternative physicians for cancer.

*Immunoglobulin* A globulin is a protein that, as its name implies, globs onto a foreign protein, marking it for attack by T-cells. Think of globulins as the scouts of the immune system that stake out the bad guys. One of the main immunoglobulins, IgA, is the primary antibody released by the walls of the mucous membranes and intestinal tract. It does its "glob-ing" in the digestive tract, binding to bad bacteria and viruses, preventing them from passing through the walls of the gut into the rest of the body.

*Transfer factor* Immune cells learn by transferring vital information from one cell to the next. This chain of command alerts the immune foot soldiers of potential troublemakers. Transfer factor makes this exchange of information possible. It is how a new mother passes her immunity onto her offspring, making the newborn's immune system smarter and better able to recognize antigens. At any age, older and wiser immune cells pass on their antibody memory to younger cells via transfer factor. Transfer factor improves the intracellular communication network. It is not unlike adding new phone lines!

> *Fibronectin* This compound makes phagocytes (immune cells that gobble up foreign proteins) more aggressive so that they weed out microbes even before they have been alerted by antibodies. Fibronectin makes the immune system more flexible: not only can it follow orders but it can also act independently to weed out problems.
>
> *Growth factors* Infants are born with an immature, or "leaky," gut that does not adequately prevent materials in the GI tract from seeping into other body tissues. It is for this reason that we can only feed breast milk or formula to young babies in the first year of life. Feeding them foreign protein can trigger a terrible allergic reaction. Growth factors in breast milk help the infant's digestive tract mature more quickly. Some growth factors also stimulate wound healing in adults.

mans and mammals. It is chock full of potent immune enhancing factors that help jumpstart the infant's immature immune system. What colostrum is to infants, it can also be to adults—a sturdy framework on which to build a better immune system. Scientists have made progress in isolating the substances in it that make it so beneficial to immune systems, both mature and immature:

All these ingredients make colostrum an excellent general immune booster for adults. I usually do not recommend using colostrum alone for acute conditions because it is primarily a long-term builder. It does not have the immediate antibacterial or antiviral punch of olive leaf extract or garlic.

(I do, however, include it with other immunotics for treatment of acute conditions.) Rather, colostrum works best when used as a tonic to promote overall health or fight chronic conditions. In particular, I have found colostrum to be excellent for chronic GI infections, including irritable bowel disorder, chronic diarrhea, Crohn's disease, ulcerative colitis, and stomach ulcers. Colostrum helps control the bacterial overgrowth typical of these problems without disturbing the normal balance of flora in the gut. I have also used colostrum to augment the treatment of *Heliobacter pylori* bacteria, a major cause of ulcers. These patients should begin taking colostrum (6–9 capsules daily) at the start of antibiotic therapy, continuing on for 2 to 3 months thereafter to prevent recurrence.

I also recommend colostrum for nonspecific immune problems. For example, if I have a patient who has had three to four different infections over the past year or two that required antibiotic therapy, I suspect that his or her immune system is not functioning properly. Colostrum gently but effectively gets the immune function back up to snuff. I also prescribe colostrum for people who need continual immune support, such as those suffering from recurrent sinus infections, the parents of young children, and the immunocompromised.

While many of the components in colostrum, such as lactoferrin and transfer factor, are sold as individual supplements, I believe that Mother Nature intended these various components to work together and that to break them apart may reduce their effectiveness.

Colostrum is safe for most people. Producers try to eliminate allergy-causing proteins from colostrum, but someone with a milk allergy may still develop mild symptoms. In this case, discontinue using it. I recommend buying colostrum from cows that are raised without pesticides, antibiotics, or growth hormones.

Some promoters claim that colostrum is an antiaging supplement that does everything from promoting muscle growth and weight loss to curing depression. Frankly, I can't vouch for it for these purposes, and I am loath to say that a compound does something that I can't scientifically verify; however, future research may well support these claims.

One final note: Many of my patients have expressed concern that taking colostrum from a cow may hurt the newborn calf. That is not true. The brands that I recommend use only a small amount of colostrum from each cow, leaving plenty to nourish the young calf.

### Cranberry

**Rx:** The immunotic for bladder and urinary tract infections.

**The Right Amount:** Range: 400–2400 mg daily. Lower dose: To prevent infections, take 2 (200 mg) capsules daily. Higher dose: At the first sign of infection, start with a loading dose of 2 capsules of cranberry extract, then take 1 capsule every 3–4 hours for up to 6 capsules daily.

Cranberry (*Vaccinium macrocarponum*) is another example of an effective folk remedy rediscovered in modern times. For years, natural healers and more enlightened physicians have advised patients with bladder and urinary tract infections to drink cranberry juice. Although no one knew why, cranberry juice seemed to control these common, troublesome infections, which affect about 20 percent of all women during their lifetime. Some thought that cranberry must work by making urine more acidic, killing the infecting bacteria. We now know that cranberry has an entirely different mode of action—and far more clever. Cranberry contains a substance that prevents the bacteria from adhering to the lining of the bladder and urinary tract, much as Teflon keeps food from sticking to a cooking pan. If the bacteria can't bond to the body, they get flushed out with the urine. Not only that, cranberry contains phytochemicals called anthocyanidins, which have natural antibiotic action.

By the way, although cranberries have gotten all the press, blueberries contain many of the same compounds. The problem with commercial cranberry juice is that it is light on juice and heavy on refined sugar. On the other hand, cranberry capsules have concentrated good stuff and none of the bad. I recommend them.

### Curcumin

**Rx:** Anti-inflammatory, antimicrobial, and antioxidant used to treat acute conditions such as hepatitis, HIV, postsurgical recovery and cancer. It also helps the body recover after strenuous physical activity.

**The Right Amount:** 500–1500 mg daily. Lower dose: take 1 or 2 (500 mg) capsules daily. Higher dose: take 3 (500 mg) capsules daily.

Curcumin is the active ingredient in turmeric (known by the botanical name *Curcuma longa*), the spice that gives yellow rice, commercial mustard preparations, and many other dishes an unmistakable yellow color. In addition to being a tasty spice, turmeric is part of the traditional system of medicine practiced in India called ayurveda. Curcumin is extracted from turmeric powder, which has potent antimicrobial properties, and is effective against several common pathogens, including fungal infections. (Interestingly, before refrigeration, turmeric was one of the spices used to preserve food.) Curcumin is one of the immunotics that I turn to to treat conditions that require strong antioxidant and anti-inflammatory action.

Curcumin has great value in treating inflammation of the liver. Long before ayurvedic healers knew how it worked, they prescribed turmeric for liver disorders. Today we know why their folk remedies worked so well. Curcumin increases intracellular glutathione levels. Glutathione, you may remember, is the primary antioxidant in the liver and is essential for immune health. Hepatitis causes levels of glutathione to plummet, resulting in severely impaired liver function. Since the body relies on liver to detoxify, poor liver function puts us at increased risk of disease.

There is some exciting preliminary research being done on cancer as well. In test tube studies, curcumin has thwarted the growth of several different types of cancer cells, and animal studies confirm that turmeric can slow the growth of tumors. Numerous studies have documented curcumin's power to inhibit the action of many different carcinogens. Curcumin is the subject of much ongoing research; scientists want to investigate whether it could be useful as a treatment for breast, skin, and colon cancer.

Given curcumin's safety, broad scope of action, and non-toxicity, I prescribe it to my cancer patients to augment their conventional therapies. Time will tell if curcumin is effective against cancer, but I have a hunch that it will help speed recovery. Others can benefit from the healing power of curcumin, too! I recommend curcumin for postsurgery recovery and after strenuous exercise—both of these can result in lower glutathione levels and inflammation.

Finally, I prescribe curcumin to patients who have AIDS or are HIV positive as an immunotic support along with antiviral drug therapy. People with AIDS often show low levels of glutathione, which undoubtedly contributes to their depressed immune function. As with cancer patients, immunotics such as curcumin can bolster compromised immune function and strengthen the effect of conventional therapy.

### Echinacea*

**Rx:** For acute conditions such as colds, flus, bronchitis, and sinus and skin infections.

**The Right Amount:** 500–4000 mg daily, for 14 days. Lower dose: take 1 dropperful of tincture or 1 (500 mg) capsule in the morning and in the afternoon. Higher dose: take 2 dropperfuls of tincture or 2 (500 mg) capsules every 2 hours for up to 4 hours.

**Special Instructions:** I recommend products that combine two different species of echinacea—*Echinacea augustifolia* and *Echinacea purpurea*. Echinacea works best when taken in small doses throughout the day.

Echinacea, a member of the daisy family, is probably the best known of all the immunotics. I have used it myself and prescribed it to my patients for more than 20 years. Although it is one of the best-selling supplements of all time, there is still great confusion and misunderstanding about it. I will try to clear up some of that here.

First, a bit of echinacea's fascinating history. Native Americans living on the Great Plains relied on echinacea to treat a wide variety of medical ailments, including coughs, colds, sore throats, infections, toothaches, snakebites, and skin wounds. They shared their knowledge with the early settlers, who quickly incorporated this herb into their natural pharmacy and introduced echinacea to Europe. In the early United States, echinacea was touted as a "blood purifier" that could cure everything from bee stings to syphilis. I'm sure *some* of that might have been true! By the nineteenth century, the Western medical establishment changed its focus and began to turn away from herbal medicine to chemotherapy—the use of chemical drugs such as sulfur, arsenic, and mercury—to treat disease. Nonetheless, echinacea retained a strong following among both physicians and patients in the United States until after World War II—a testament to its potency. When antibiotics arrived, it was abandoned. Though forgotten in the United States, echinacea was still used widely in Germany, where it prospered as a treatment and as the subject of scientific study.

In the 1970s, the growing environmental movement sweeping the United States sparked a renewed interest in natural remedies such as echinacea. In fact, I think that echinacea may have even helped start the boom. Health food stores began to crop up around the country. At that time echinacea was not sold in convenient capsules, tablets, or ready-made teas as it is today. If you wanted to use echinacea, you had to buy the dried herb and make your own tea or extract; this discouraged many potential users, who were too sick for such effort.

By the 1980s, two major world events greatly enhanced the popularity of this once forgotten herb. First, the AIDS epidemic created a surge of interest in substances—natural or otherwise—that could enhance immune function. Americans soon became aware of European studies that suggested that echinacea was effective as an immunostimulant. Second, the development of antibiotic-resistant bugs also accelerated the search for alternative natural infection fighters. Both of these events put the medical community on notice that conventional infection fighting could fail. It opened up the possibility of high-level American scientific exploration of immune-enhancing compounds. By the 1990s, various forms of echinacea (capsules, tinctures, teas, extracts) were cropping up everywhere, from drugstores to discount stores to supermarkets, and even in doctors' offices. Echinacea promoters asserted that it should be taken every day for overall immune health, a contention with which I disagree, as you'll see.

First, let me clear up the primary misconception about echinacea. Countless numbers of people take echinacea daily in the belief that it will *prevent* colds and flus. This is simply not true. I know this not only from personal observation but also from a study published in the *Archives of Family Medicine;* echinacea is no better at preventing colds than a placebo (a sugar pill). Press accounts of this study compounded the misunderstandings, concluding that echinacea doesn't work at all. That, too, is incorrect. Echinacea works quite well, but only for acute illnesses. In other words, you should take echinacea when you feel sick, not when you feel well.

Numerous studies document that echinacea does indeed boost immune function. In particular, it enhances phagocytosis, the process by which immune cells gobble up and destroy bacteria and other foreign particles. It also provides immune cells with a powerful weapon to fight against infection: a potent free radical called superoxide anion. In an interesting study, reported in *Science News* (March 27, 1999), a researcher at the University of Florida in Gainesville gave echinacea to 10 male college students for four days. The researcher then separated out immune cells collected from the volunteers and subjected them to a technique that mimics attack by an infectious agent. After the echinacea treatment, the immune cells produced much higher levels of superoxide anion. Keep in mind that you would not want to produce higher levels of this free radical all the time—in fact, it could be harmful—but it's a good thing to have around when your body is fighting a cold or flu bug.

The Commission E of the German Institute for Drugs and Medical Devices (their version of our FDA) has approved echinacea as a nonprescriptive therapy for colds, chronic infections, and influenza. A recent Swedish study involved 199 patients who took either echinacea or a placebo at the first sign of a cold. Both patients and their physicians evaluated the effectiveness of treatment based on 12 common cold symptoms. The physicians reported that they felt echinacea was effective in 68 percent of the patients. Patients rated it even higher—78 percent considered it effective in reducing symptoms.

In my personal, purely anecdotal opinion, echinacea does not work as well or as consistently as it did 20 years ago. When I first began using and recommending echinacea, it worked liked magic for colds and respiratory bugs. Today, it doesn't seem to pack the same punch, and there are two possible reasons why. First, people overusing echinacea may diminish its effectiveness in their bodies. In other words, once your body gets used to it, it doesn't elicit as strong a response. Second, some brands of echinacea may not have all the potency they advertise. Be sure to buy standardized extract, which guarantees potency—from a reliable manufacturer.

Echinacea has one side effect: it can produce mild upset stomach in some people. The chemical structure of echinacea is a complex carbohydrate similar to fiber, which can cause gas and bloating. If it bothers you, switch to a different immunotic.

Despite these caveats, I still recommend echinacea either alone or in combination with other immunotics to help shake off a cold or speed up recovery from the flu. When it works, it works well; but treat it carefully.

## Elderberry

**Rx:** The herb to take at the first sign of flu.

**The Right Amount:** Range: 2–4 teaspoons daily. For acute conditions: Take 1 teaspoon of elderberry extract every 3–4 hours for up to 10 days.

Since the days of Hippocrates, European blackberries (known by the botanical name of *Sambucus nigra*) have been used as a folk remedy for colds, flus, and respiratory infections. Recently, researchers at Hadassah University Medical Center in Jerusalem unraveled the science behind this folk cure. They discovered that specific proteins in elderberry can help prevent the flu virus from replicating, reducing flu symptoms and speeding recovery. Unlike bacteria, viruses cannot survive on their own and need to hijack other cells to reproduce. A flu virus enters a cell by puncturing the cell membrane with tiny spikes of an enzyme designed to destroy the cell membrane. Once inside, the virus uses the cell's own machinery to reproduce itself. Elderberry knocks out the flu virus in two important ways. First, it binds to the viral spikes, preventing them from piercing the cell membrane. Second, it inhibits the chemical action of the enzyme designed to weaken the membrane. The end result is that elderberry makes it difficult, if not impossible, for the flu virus to reproduce.

In 1992 Israeli scientists patented a specially designed elderberry product called Sambucol, which combined elderberry extract with other virus-fighting compounds. They had a perfect opportunity to test it during the winter of 1992–93, when a flu epidemic broke out in a kibbutz in southern Israel. The researchers gave flu victims Sambucol or a placebo in a double blind study. Within 24 hours, 20 percent of the elderberry-treated group showed dramatic improvement in fever, muscle pain, and respiratory symptoms. By the second day of treatment, 75 percent showed significant improvement, and by the third day, 90 percent felt markedly better. In the placebo group, only 8 percent felt better within 24 hours, 16 percent felt better in 48 hours, and the rest took six days to improve. Clearly, Sambucol made a difference in recovery time. And that's not all elderberry can do: further research at Hadassah Hospital showed that elderberry is effective against certain cancer cells in test tube studies and can boost immune response.

I include elderberry extract in my formula to treat acute flu symptoms. It works even better in combination with other immunotics.

### Flaxseed Oil*

**Rx:** A terrific immunotic for everybody . . . but especially for school-aged children and teenagers.

**The Right Amount:** Range: sprinkle 1–3 tablespoons of ground flaxseed on food daily. Ground flaxseed also tastes great! Try it on yogurt, cereal, or in a protein shake.

Low-fat diets have become a way of life for many Americans, who have been led to believe that cutting back on fat will save them from cancer, obesity, and heart disease. This all-or-nothing approach is only half right. Although some types of fat (primarily the saturated fat found in meat and dairy products) may promote disease, you need fat in your diet to stay healthy. In fact, some types of fat are critical for a healthy immune system. Called essential fatty acids, they are sorely lacking in our modern diet and especially in the diets of children.

Essential fatty acids are needed everywhere in the body. They are the major components of cell membranes. And hormones—the chemical messengers that run every body system—cannot be produced without them. Since the body cannot make essential fatty acids on its own, it must get them through food.

The body uses two types of essential fatty acids: omega-6 and omega-3. Some omega-3 fatty acids are converted in the body into eicosapentaenoic acid (EPA) and docosahexanoic acid (DHA). Both EPA and DHA are very important for children's physical and emotional health. A terrific immune booster, EPA increases natural killer-cell activity while decreasing prostaglandins, the hormonelike substances that promote inflammation. Children must have DHA for proper brain development. Low levels of DHA have been linked to depression, alcoholism, violent behavior, and learning disorders in children. Your child needs omega-3 fatty acids for his or her long-term health as well. Several test tube studies have shown that omega-3 fatty acids can shrink cancerous tumors, and preliminary human studies suggest that these fats may have a potent inhibitory effect on breast cancer cells. Omega-3 fatty acids can also reduce high blood cholesterol and triglyceride levels.

Omega-6 fatty acids are found in nuts, seeds, avocados, and many cooking oils; we tend to get an adequate supply of them in our diet—if not too much! Omega-3 fatty acids are found in cold water fatty fish (like salmon, tuna, sardines, and mackerel), some seeds, and grains. Our hunter-gatherer ancestors had an omega-3 to omega-6 fatty acid ratio of about 1 to 2. Today, the ratio is about 1 to 24, meaning nearly five times less in our diet. Many researchers believe that the decline in omega-3 fatty acids in our diet increases the risk of heart disease and cancer. Our modern diet makes it difficult to get enough omega-3 fatty acids from food alone. Even if you eat a lot of fish, you may still be deficient—omega-3 fatty acids accumulate in the skin, which many people do not eat. Furthermore, they can be destroyed by freezing or during cooking.

Flaxseed is one of the best sources of omega-3 fatty acids—even better than some fish. In fact, it used to be a mainstay of the human diet. About 8,500 years ago, our hunter-gatherer ancestors ate flax along with other wild grasses. Today, flaxseed oil is making a comeback and is now being sold in health food stores around the country. However, flaxseed is not easy to use. Notoriously unstable, unless properly processed, it can turn rancid quickly. Capsules may be hard for children to swallow. One alternative is to use ground flaxseed. You can purchase whole or ground flaxseed from a health food store. Sprinkle it on your children's cereal, yogurt, and salad or even inside their peanut butter and jelly sandwich. It is flavorless and odorless and very easy to get down.

By the way, there's no reason why everybody in the family shouldn't take a daily dose of flaxseed!

### Garlic*

**Rx:** Good for many ills, but especially effective in treating gut problems.

**The Right Amount:** Take 300–900 mg of dried garlic extract daily (equivalent to 1–3 cloves). Lower dose: take 1 (300 mg) capsule daily. Higher dose: take 3 (300 mg) capsules daily.

For more than 20 years, garlic has been a mainstay of my medical practice. Although garlic works for a wide range of ailments (you might already be using it to boost your heart health) it is my immunotic of choice for problems related to the gut, especially yeast overgrowth, stomach bugs, and recurrent bowel problems. I recommend it in connection with other immunotics for acute colds and flus and as a cancer preventer.

Garlic can be eaten fresh (it is most potent raw) or taken in tablet form. But not all garlic supplements are the same: some processing destroys many of garlic's benefits. If you don't go the fresh route, use only dried whole garlic. Many of my patients eat one fresh garlic clove—*not* a whole bulb—daily to prevent infection. Take 1 garlic clove (about the size of your thumb) and crush it with the flat side of a knife. Wait for 10 minutes to activate the enzymes that liberate the disease-fighting ingredients. Before eating, mix a teaspoon of honey into the crushed garlic to make it more palatable. Enjoy. Many of my patients swear by this, especially during cold and flu season. By the way, I recommend that everyone in the family do this, for obvious reasons.

Used as food and medicine for more than five thousand years, garlic is a member of the lily family, which includes its close relatives onions, chives, and leeks. Long before the dawn of modern medicine, physicians recognized the powerful healing properties of these vegetables. (And chefs recognized the taste!)

Even the Egyptians prized garlic for its health benefits. King Tut went to the next world with six dried garlic cloves in his tomb. On the other end of the social spectrum, Egyptians fed extra rations of garlic to their slaves while they were building the pyramids because they believed that it promoted endurance and health. In fact, according to the Bible, when the Israelites were wandering through the Sinai dessert after their escape from Egypt, they bitterly complained about missing those garlic rations. The ancient Greeks and

Romans also used garlic as a tonic for health and vitality. European crusaders brought garlic back from the Middle East, introducing garlic to Europe. Just in time, too. Chewing on garlic probably saved the lives of many a saintly monk tending to the legions of people sick with bubonic plague. Actually, this makes a lot of sense. Whole garlic is one of the strongest antibiotics in the natural pharmacy. But when it comes to plague, garlic's secret weapon is its smell. The plague was spread throughout Europe by fleas living on such animals as rats. If you eat a lot of garlic, its pungent odor leeches from the gut into the blood and out through the skin. Repelled by this odor, insects avoid contact with the reeking humans or animals. This could explain why garlic eaters avoided contracting the plague. In fact, some organic farmers still use garlic as a natural insecticide today.

Louis Pasteur, the first scientist to espouse the germ theory of disease, reported that garlic could kill or stop the growth of various types of bacteria grown in culture, a fact that was later confirmed by modern scientists. While working as a physician in Africa, Albert Schweitzer used garlic to treat cholera, typhus, and amoebic dysentery. In both world wars, garlic poultices were used on the battlefield to treat war wounds and were given orally for dysentery. But the battlefield is a dirty place, and death from infection was rampant until the introduction of penicillin. Like other immunotics, garlic works best for common, mild, everyday infections. Garlic illustrates the whole point of this book: If we use immunotics for the run-of-the-mill bugs, we can save antibiotics for the truly life-threatening ones.

After the discovery of antibiotics, garlic, no longer valued for its medicinal properties in the industrialized world, remained popular only in the kitchen. When it became apparent that antibiotics were not the answer to all of our ills, scientists once again became interested in natural remedies like garlic. They were surprised by what they found: garlic contains a veritable pharmacy of healing compounds:

- Garlic provides a natural blood thinner called ajoene, which prevents blood clots.
- Garlic is an excellent source of the mineral selenium, important in the creation of glutathione.
- Allicin, one of the active ingredients responsible for garlic's health benefits, has antimicrobial properties and effectively controls yeast overgrowth, parasites, disease-causing bacteria, and viruses.
- Garlic boosts NK cell activity.
- Garlic may inhibit the growth of many different types of cancer cells, according to test tube and animal studies.
- Garlic prevents cancer-causing breaks in DNA strands that are caused by free radicals that can promote cancer.

Much of the recent attention given to garlic centers around its potential use as a cancer fighter. According to a study sponsored by the United States National Cancer Institute of about four thousand people in China and Italy, those who ate the most garlic (and other allium vegetables) had a significantly lower risk of developing stomach cancer than those who did not. Further research performed at Pennsylvania State University showed that garlic inhibits the formation of nitrosamines, powerful carcinogens formed in the stomach from the food additive sodium nitrate. (Nitrates are used to cure meats such as hot dogs and bacon. If you must eat a hot dog on the Fourth of July, be sure to eat it with garlic!) Recently, researchers at Memorial Sloan-Kettering Cancer Research Center found that garlic may help prevent and treat prostate cancer, the second most common cancer in men (following skin cancer.) When they exposed prostate cancer cells grown in culture dishes to a sulphur compound found in garlic, the garlic compound significantly slowed down their growth. Interestingly, they found that garlic helped control the excess amounts of the form of testosterone that triggers the growth of prostate tumors. I have a hunch that the more we find out about this ancient remedy, the more applications we will find for it today.

Several studies confirm that garlic kills the amoebas that cause amoebic dysentery. I recommend it highly as a treatment for stomach bugs because, unlike antibiotics, it kills the bad organisms without causing further stomach upset.

Since the widespread use of antibiotics and steroid drugs (which are immune suppressants), virulent yeast infections have been on the rise. Yeast are hardy organisms. Any drug that can control them often has very unpleasant side effects for the human host. Garlic, on the other hand, can wipe out many types of yeast infections, and without unpleasant side effects. In fact, a student at Cambridge University reports that garlic juice is equal in potency to two commonly prescribed antifungal drugs. Not surprisingly, garlic has long been used as an antifungal treatment by healers in tropical countries, where fungal infections are common.

**Grapefruit Seed Extract***

**Rx:** For both acute intestinal bugs and to prevent traveler's diarrhea.

**The Right Amount:** Range: 10 to 30 drops of extract daily—always dilute extract in 8 ounces of water or juice. Take 10 drops of extract in 8 ounces of liquid up to 3 times daily. Do not use in the nausea or vomiting stage.

Grapefruit seed extract (also called citrus seed extract) is a natural antiseptic that I use primarily for intestinal problems such as traveler's diarrhea or parasitic infections. It is a MUST HAVE for anyone traveling to a country where water and sanitary conditions are less than optimal. The highly concentrated liquid extract must be diluted in a glass of water or juice. Grapefruit seed extract is strong medicine and should never be used full strength. When diluted with liquid, however, it is perfectly safe. Do not use grapefruit seed extract on your skin—it can be quite irritating. The food industry uses grapefruit seed extract as a food preservative to protect fruits and vegetables from fungal and other infections.

**Green Tea Extract***

**Rx:** For people who are at greater risk of developing cancer due to heredity, medical history, or lifestyle. Also of benefit to people with chronic hepatitis.

**The Right Amount:** Green tea extract is sold in capsules or tablets in varying strengths. I recommend 1000 mg daily.

For thousands of years, real tea (not the herbal kind) has been made from the tea plant, *Camellia sinsensis.* This evergreen plant produces three kinds of tea: green tea, oolong, and black tea. Unlike the other varieties of tea, green tea is unfermented, while black tea and oolong tea achieve their particular strength and character through curing. All tea contains antioxidant compounds called polyphenols, but the polyphenols in green tea are believed to be the most potent. In fact, under some situations, green tea polyphenols have a greater antioxidant action than either vitamins C or E.

Studies show that green tea drinkers have lower rates of stomach, lung, esophageal, colon, and pancreatic cancer than those who don't. In fact, population studies have definitively linked green tea consumption to a dramatically reduced cancer risk. In particular, green tea polyphenols can inhibit the formation of nitrosamine—a nasty food carcinogen I mentioned earlier—quench free radicals, and protect LDL or bad cholesterol from oxidative damage (which leads to heart disease.)

Green tea is most effective in high doses. That is, the more tea you drink, the greater the reduction in cancer risk. One recent study showed that Japanese women who drank 10 cups of green tea daily had a significantly lower risk of breast cancer than those who drank less. Although green tea contains half the caffeine of coffee, 10 cups of tea is still equivalent to four to five cups of coffee, a hefty dose of caffeine. The caffeine in green tea may have a synergistic effect with the polyphenols, enhancing their antioxidant action. So my advice is, unless you can't tolerate caffeine, you can safely drink two cups of caffeinated green tea daily. An easier way to get your green tea is with extracts, available in capsule or tablet form.

> **IP-6 \***
>
> **Rx:**  A potent immunotic for serious conditions such as cancer, hepatitis, and HIV, when used along with other conventional therapies.
>
> **The Right Amount:**  Range: each capsule contains 400 mg IP-6 with 110 mg inositol. I recommend 4 to 12 capsules daily.

IP-6 is a new supplement that combines inositol, a common substance extracted from food, with phosphate to create a natural chemical called inositol hexaphosphate, or phytic acid. When joined together these two nutrients turn into a powerful cancer-fighting combo. I recommend IP-6 for my patients with cancer who have undergone conventional treatment and want to do all they can to prevent a recurrence. Despite its power, I do not believe that IP-6 by itself can cure an existing cancer. However, it can hasten recovery and may even prevent cancer in the first place.

Among its many actions, IP-6 enhances the activity of NK cells, making it a useful adjuvant treatment not only for cancer but also for other serious immune-destroying illnesses such as hepatitis or AIDS.

IP-6 is a more concentrated form of the same phytic acid that is found in some high-fiber foods, such as rice, wheat, legumes, and soybeans. For years, researchers noted a link between high-fiber diets and a reduced risk of developing certain types of cancer. Not all forms of fiber, however, appeared to be equal when it came to preventing cancer. In fact, population studies suggested that diets high in two specific grains—rice and wheat—offered the *most* protection against cancer. Diets rich in other forms of fiber, such as corn or oat bran, were not nearly as effective. Rice and wheat are the two grains that are highest in phytic acid, and this information piqued the curiosity of scientists.

Much of the work on phytic acid has been performed by Abulkalam M. Shamsuddin, professor of pathology at the University of Maryland School of Medicine. He details his work in his fascinating book *IP6: Nature's Revolutionary Cancer-Fighter;* after reading it, it would be difficult for even the most skeptical of physicians not to take IP-6 seriously. Inositol—one of the building blocks of phytic acid—is no stranger to the human body. A sugarlike molecule essential for many different cellular functions, it is ubiquitous throughout our cells. In particular, inositol is a signal transduction agent, which simply means that it "turns on" and "turns off" genes. IP-6, a more efficient form of inositol, appears to turn on our cancer-fighting genes while turning off the cancer-promoting ones.

Cancer is the result of genes gone haywire. All cancers involve the abnormal growth of cells, and that is regulated by genes. Normally, our cells reproduce and die in an orderly fashion. Our genes regulate cell birth and death—known as the cell cycle—by knowing precisely when to activate growth and when to suppress it. Cancer happens when the normal cell cycle is thrown out of whack. The cancer process begins when a cell mutates and begins to reproduce wildly. It doesn't happen overnight; in fact, it can take years for a cell to turn cancerous. Once it does, these bad cells can invade healthy cells, robbing them of their nutrients to feed the cancer. A specific protein (called P53) within each cell functions as an internal brake on growth. When exposed to a cancer agent, however, P53 can lose some of its punch, making it unable to halt the uncontrolled cell growth. And that can lead to cancer. One way IP-6 works is by making P53 more effective, restoring the normal cell cycle. So strong is its effect that IP-6 can help precancerous cells revert to normal. In other words, it can turn a potentially bad cell good before it can do its dirty work.

Like other immunotics, IP-6 also has a direct effect on the immune system by boosting NK cell activity: While it is preventing destructive cell growth, it is giving the immune system the ammunition it needs to weed out potential cancers.

Why take a supplement when you can get the same thing from food? Although it's true that population studies confirm that eating a diet rich in phytic acid helps reduce the risk of cancer, keep in mind that these studies are based on long-term eating habits. I am a firm believer that eating low levels of cancer-fighting compounds over a long period of time will have a beneficial effect. But when you're sick, you may need something stronger and faster. Dr. Shamsuddin tested the cancer-fighting potential of IP-6 versus a high-fiber diet on rats that were fed a carcinogen known to induce mammary breast cancer. He fed one group of rats a high-fiber diet rich in phytic acid for two weeks prior to administration of the carcinogen. The rats were given three versions of the diet: 5 percent, 10 percent, or 20 percent bran (equal to a human dose of 500–1000 mg of IP-6). A second group of rats was given the same diet and carcinogen, but IP-6 was put in their drinking water (equal to a human dose of about

500–1000 mg daily). After 29 weeks, he found that the rats eating the fiber-rich diet showed a modest reduction in tumor incidence, but there was little statistical difference among the three groups. The 5 percent group showed a 16.7 percent reduction; the 10 percent group showed a 14.6 percent reduction, and the 20 percent group showed an 11.4 percent reduction. In scientific terms, there was little statistical difference among the three groups. The results were far more dramatic for the group given IP-6 in their drinking water—they showed a 33.5 percent reduction in tumor incidence and 48.8 percent fewer tumors per animal, a very strong statistically significant showing. Similar studies have shown that IP-6 can also inhibit colon cancer in animals. The combination of the population studies and these animal studies suggests that IP-6 may work as well in humans. Indeed, we know from anecdotal reports that it is helpful for many different types of cancer. A carefully conducted human trial would answer many of the unanswered questions.

IP-6 and similar immunotics fill an important gap in medicine. All too often, after patients have undergone cancer treatment, their cancer specialists tell them to come back in a year to see if the treatment has worked. Sadly, they do not give them any information on the important steps they could be taking to reduce the odds of recurrence. IP-6 can be a useful tool, along with eating the right diet and living a healthy lifestyle, for patients who want to do all they can to stay cancer free.

Should people who are at high risk of developing cancer consider taking IP-6? Personally, I think it's a good idea. I also recommend IP-6 for some patients with hepatitis C who are at added risk of developing liver cancer.

**7 KETO DHEA***

**Rx:** Tonic for an aging immune system.
**The Right Amount:** Range: 25–50 mg daily. Lower dose: take 1 (25 mg) capsule daily. Higher dose: Take 2 (25 mg) capsules daily.

*DHEA* is short for dehydroepiandrosterone. Similar to estrogen and testosterone, DHEA is a steroid, a type of hormone found in abundance in the human body; it is produced by the adrenal glands, the brain, and the skin. It is, in fact, the most abundant steroid in the human body. As with many things, levels of DHEA decline with age, dropping 2 percent a year from age 20 on. By age 80, we only have 15 percent of the DHEA we had at 25. By age 90, it's all gone. The drop in DHEA coincides with many of the symptoms we associate with aging, including the measurable drop in immune function that typifies immunosenescence. Many physicians and researchers believe that the drop in DHEA is in part responsible for the physical and even mental decline that we have long associated with aging. Restoring DHEA to youthful levels could help reverse some of the telltale signs of aging, including immunosenescence.

DHEA breaks down in the body into two other hormones, estrogen and testosterone. Therefore, DHEA offers many of the same positive effects of hormone replacement. Unfortunately, it may offer the negative as well. Hormone replacement therapy has been implicated in an increased risk of certain cancers. In addition, some women find that DHEA in particular can have too much of a testosterone effect, including the growth of facial hair.

Recently, a new type of DHEA has been brought to market called 7 KETO DHEA, which has many of the beneficial effects of DHEA but none of the side effects. I recommend 7 KETO DHEA to my patients who are over 45 and who are beginning to show signs of immunosenescence.

Hundreds of human and animal studies have confirmed that DHEA replacement therapy can have a beneficial effect on immune function, in several key ways:

- In a recent study conducted by Omid Khorran, a professor of medicine at the University of San Diego, nine healthy older men were given DHEA supplements for five months. Dr. Khorran found that DHEA stimulated both the production of T-cells and NK cell activity, which are both essential for fighting infection.

- DHEA appears to help restore balance to the immune system. Preliminary studies suggest that it is useful in treating autoimmune diseases such as lupus. In a study of postmenopausal women at the University of Tennessee, researchers found that women taking DHEA experienced a rise in the activity of NK cells and a decline in a hormonelike substance that has been linked causally to autoimmune diseases and other diseases of aging.

- Vaccinations are not always as effective in older people as they are in younger ones. Several studies have shown that DHEA can help older immune systems produce antibodies from vaccinations with the same vigor as a younger immune system.

There are other benefits to DHEA that go beyond its role in the immune system: It makes people feel better. In a groundbreaking study of 13 men and 17 women conducted at the University of San Diego, those taking DHEA reported a "remarkable increase in perceived physical and psychological well-being for both men and women." My own patients have told me the same thing.

Before I prescribe 7 KETO DHEA to my patients, first I take a blood test to see if they are low in DHEA, just like I do when prescribing estrogen. If the blood test confirms my suspicions, I recommend 7 KETO DHEA supplements. The blood test should be repeated every three to six months after beginning 7 KETO DHEA to check that DHEA is within normal limits. Since, in rare cases, DHEA can alter liver function, I also do periodic liver enzyme checks on my patients taking this hormone.

### Lemon Balm*

**Rx:** Good overall immune booster, antiviral, and topical anesthetic for cold sores.

**The Right Amount:** Apply the ointment to the infected area 4 to 6 times daily.

For hundreds of years, lemon balm (*Melissa officinalis*) has held a key place in the herbal pharmacy for treating stomach upset, insomnia, and nerve pain. I use it to treat a very modern problem: herpes. Lemon balm is a rich source of polyphenol compounds, which effectively battle the herpes virus. You have no doubt heard of herpes as an infamous sexually transmitted disease. However, variations of the same virus (Herpes Simplex 1) are responsible for those troublesome cold sores that also crop up. German physicians share my faith in lemon balm. It is a widely prescribed treatment for both genital herpes and cold sores.

### L-Glutamine*

**Rx:** For athletes under physical stress, people with chronic gut problems, and those recovering from surgery.

**The Right Amount:** Range: 5 to 15 grams of powder daily (1 teaspoon is 5 grams). Lower dose: mix ½–1 teaspoon powder in a small amount of water 1 or 2 times daily. Higher dose: mix 1 teaspoon powder in small amount of water 3 times daily.

**Special Instructions:** L-glutamine is also available in capsules, but you would have to take more than 20 capsules to meet my recommended dose. The powder is more efficient and economical.

The building blocks of protein, amino acids are an essential component of the human body, and L-glutamine is the most abundant of them. L-glutamine comprises more than half of the total amount of amino acids within the body and 60 percent of the total amino acids within muscle. L-glutamine, among all amino acids, is required for a well-functioning immune system; it is necessary for the production of lymphocytes, and the activation of macrophages depends on supplies of it. In fact, I've heard L-glutamine described as "fuel" for the immune system. It is one of the key immunotics I recommend to endurance athletes or vigorous exercisers.

Endurance athletes are especially vulnerable to upper respiratory tract infections after prolonged training or competition. Although mild to moderate exercise can boost immune function, intense physical training can dampen it. The measurable decline in immune cell activity after severe physical exertion can last for days. There are several reasons for this. First, during intense exercise, the body consumes oxygen at a much higher rate. High oxygen use leads to more free radicals, which in turn depletes immune-boosting antioxidants. Second, although glutamine levels rise after moderate physical activity, they plummet after intense exercise. When the body is under physical stress, it quickly depletes its store of glutamine. Several studies have reported that glutamine supplements reduce the incidence of infections reported by athletes after strenuous physical activity. Glutamine also helped the athlete's immune system recover faster after exertion.

German scientists recently reported that glutamine has a protective effect on the lining of the gut. In particular, it can help preserve the integrity of the mucosal cells of the intestines during radiation and chemotherapy, which under the best of circumstances can often cause damage to healthy tissues and organs. I include glutamine in my Immunotics program for people with chronic gut problems, with very good results. After glutamine treatment, patients report less gas, bloating, and abdominal pain. On another front, I also recommend glutamine to patients after surgery because it has been shown to prevent the muscle wasting that can occur during periods of prolonged bed rest.

Asian healers have extolled the healing powers of mush-

**Medicinal Mushrooms: Maitake, Reishi, and Shiitake\***

**Rx:** These three Asian mushrooms are terrific immune boosters. Choose the mushroom that best suits your needs. Shiitake works for people at high risk for colds and flus. Reishi can help the body cope better with physical or emotional stress. The most potent of the three, maitake, is my choice for cancer prevention and chronic hepatitis. It is also the most expensive.

**The Right Amount:** The right dose will depend on which mushroom product you use and for what condition you are using it.

| | |
|---|---|
| *Shiitake:* | Take 1 (500 mg) capsule daily. |
| *Reishi:* | Take 1 (500 mg) capsule daily. |
| *Maitake D-Fraction:* | Take 1 dropperful up to 3 times daily. (Although this is the most expensive of the three, it is a highly concentrated form of maitake.) |

rooms, using them for thousands of years to treat a wide variety of ailments. Only recently have we Western physicians discovered what these traditional healers have known for centuries: mushrooms can be strong medicine.

In particular, science has focused on three specific types of mushrooms: shiitake (*Lentinan edodes*), reishi (*Ganoderma lucidum*) and maitake (*Grifola frondosa*). Shiitake and maitake are used in Asian cooking. But beyond their delicious flavor, mushrooms are a great source of beta glucans, molecules made up of repeating units of glucose (sugar). When beta glucans bind to NK cells, T-cells, and macrophages, they elicit a strong immune response, measurably increasing their activity. No one knows precisely why immune cells respond to beta glucans, but some scientists think that beta glucans "trick" immune cells into thinking they are under attack. Since mushrooms are basically molds, and molds are a type of fungi, perhaps our cells believe that the harmless mushrooms are dangerous pathogens.

Each type of mushroom has a slightly different form of beta glucan, but the particular chemical structure of maitake may make it the most potent immune enhancer of all the Asian mushrooms. (Of course, you can get some benefit by eating mushrooms, which I recommend, but they do not pack the same punch as using a more concentrated extract.)

**Maitake: For Cancer**

In Japanese, *maitake* means *dancing mushroom,* because legend has it that when mushroom hunters found this rare delight in the mountains of western Japan, they would dance for joy. Recent studies suggest that there is a lot to be joyful about. Maitake is approved by the Japanese government as an adjuvant therapy for cancer. It ameliorates many of the ill effects of chemotherapy and radiation, such as nausea and extreme fatigue. Chemotherapy, in the process of killing cancer cells, also wipes out NK cells. Unfortunately, NK cells are the very cells that prevent cancer cells from spreading. Animal studies performed in Japan show that maitake extract can shrink tumors in mice as well as a standard chemotherapy drug. Moreover, the combination of maitake and the chemotherapy drug worked even better than either substance alone. Human studies in Japan confirm that maitake can boost the effectiveness of standard chemotherapy for many different types of cancer. Studies underway in the United States, sponsored by the Cancer Treatment Centers of America, suggest that maitake can reduce the nasty side effects of chemotherapy.

A word of caution: Immunotics like maitake must always be used in combination with a standard cancer treatment. I am not convinced that any immunotic is strong enough to wipe out an existing cancer on its own. These supplements are best used to enhance the effect of the primary treatment, while fortifying the immune system to prevent a recurrence. As noted earlier, I strongly believe that cancer prevention—especially among people who have a history of the disease—is a sorely neglected area in medicine. Therefore, I often prescribe a specially prepared maitake extract (marketed under the name *Maitake D-Fraction*) for my patients who really need strong immune support, specifically those with cancer or a family history of cancer.

### Reishi: Stress Buster

Reishi is the mushroom of choice for people under extreme physical or emotional stress. It was known as the "medicine of kings" in Japan for more than two thousand years; Asian healers have prescribed reishi for numerous ailments, from allergies to high blood pressure and insomnia to diabetes. In particular, reishi has a long tradition of reducing stress and enhancing stamina. I recommend it for endurance athletes and during times of intense emotional stress.

### Shiitake: Immune Boost for High Risk

Shiitake mushrooms have become popular in the United States because of their delicious, hearty flavor. What you may not know is that an extract of shiitake, lentinan, is approved as a treatment for cancer in Japan. Shiitake extract is also being studied as a potential treatment for prostate cancer at the University of California, Davis, Cancer Center in Sacramento. Like reishi, shiitake has also been used to treat high cholesterol and overall immune weakness. I recommend shiitake to people who are in high-risk situations (hospital workers, parents of school-aged children, etc.) who need a potent immune boost but do not require the more expensive maitake.

## MGN-3 *

**Rx:** A potent immunotic for cancer and HIV.
**The Right Amount:** Take 1000–3000 mg daily. Lower dose: take 4 (250 mg) capsules daily. Higher dose— take 4 (250 mg) capsules 3 times daily.
**Special Instructions:** I recommend the lower dose to prevent cancer for people at high risk of developing it, and the higher dose for those who are undergoing cancer treatment or are HIV positive.

The natural pharmacy is filled with potent immunotics, but it takes a smart and persistent person to find them. A case in point is MGN-3, one of the newest immunotics on the market. MGN-3 combines modified rice bran extract with shiitake mushrooms. In scientific terms, MGN-3 is an arabinoxylane, a molecule composed of several different simple sugars found in food. Although similar to beta glucan, arabinoxylane has a slightly different mode of action. A much denser and more complex molecule than a beta glucan, arabinoxylane binds to cells differently, which in turn will trigger different reactions.

Mamdooh Ghoneum, one of the foremost authorities on NK cells and one of the first researchers to document that stress dampens NK cell activity, developed MGN-3 and has gone to great lengths to establish its scientific underpinnings. Dr. Ghoneum established that MGN-3 can significantly boost NK cell activity, a matter of particular importance to cancer patients. For this reason, I prescribe MGN-3 (or another strong NK activator) to my patients in cancer treatment. It typically works well . . . very well. Based on the experience of my patients, within two weeks of taking MGN-3, at least half of them show a doubling of NK cell activity. (As I said before, not every immunotic works for everybody. It's important to have a variety of immunotics to choose from so that you can find the one that works the best for you.)

Test tube studies have shown that MGN-3, in addition to its NK effects, has potent anticancer activity and can slow the growth of several different types of tumor cells. Not only that, it has direct antiviral action, increasing the production of virus-busting gamma-interferon.

Dr. Ghoneum tested MGN-3 on 27 patients with advanced

cancer: seven breast cancer, seven prostate, eight multiple myeloma, three leukemia, and two cervical. After undergoing conventional cancer therapy, the patients were given 3000 mg of MGN-3 daily for six months. At the beginning of the study, as might be expected, nearly all of the patients had low NK cell activity. Two weeks after treatment began, however, all of the patients showed a significant rise in NK activity, with increases ranging from 154–332 percent for breast cancer, 100–275 percent for cervical cancer, 174–385 percent for prostate cancer, 100–240 percent for leukemia, and 100–537 percent for multiple myeloma. NK cell activity continued to get stronger throughout the six-month test period.

In another study, published in the *International Journal of Immunotherapy,* Dr. Ghoneum tested MGN-3 on 11 cancer patients with advanced malignancies: 3 prostatic, 3 ovarian, 3 with multiple myeloma, and 2 with breast cancer. At the end of two weeks of treatment, 9 out of 11 patients showed a healthy increase in NK cell activity.

The fact that NK cell activity improved so dramatically does not mean that these patients are cured, but it does show that their immune systems have a better chance of fighting off the cancers. Some of the patients in these studies fared surprisingly well and went into remission. There's no way of knowing whether this would have happened without the MGN-3, but given its safety, my feeling is, why not try it?

Dr. Ghoneum has also tested MGN-3 on patients with HIV. As you may know, HIV results in a decline in NK cell activity and a sharp drop in two types of T-cells, CD4 and CD8. Dr. Ghoneum found that MGN-3 fights AIDS in two ways. It inhibits HIV replication, hampering the ability of the virus to spread, and it helps maintain T-cell activity. In his study, published in *Biochemical and Biophysical Research Communications,* he noted: "These studies demonstrated that MGN-3 has strong anti-HIV activity and may be of value in combination therapy in the treatment of HIV-1 infected patients." Once again, I'm not suggesting this is a cure for AIDS, nor am I suggesting abandoning conventional therapy, but MGN-3 may help slow down the progress of the virus, keeping people healthier for a longer period.

MGN-3 is nontoxic: very safe, with no side effects. MGN-3 is more expensive than the typical immunotic but worth it when you really need it.

### NAC

**Rx:** Great for respiratory problems, sinus infections, colds, and flu.

**The Right Amount:** Range: 1000–3000 mg daily. Lower dose: take 2 (500 mg) capsules daily. Higher dose: take 2 (500 mg) capsules 3 times daily.

Keep a bottle of NAC in your medicine cabinet and take it at the first sign of a cold or flu! I swear by it for chest colds and nasty coughs. It will lessen the severity of your symptoms and speed up your recovery.

NAC (short for N-acetyl-cysteine) is the acetylated form of the amino acid cysteine. Although relatively unknown to the public, NAC is not new in medicine. For more than two decades, this natural substance has been used in emergency rooms to treat acetaminophen poisoning. Acetaminophen is a safe drug for most people when taken at the recommended doses, but in high doses it poisons the liver by depleting the levels of glutathione. If high doses of NAC are given within eight hours after an acetaminophen overdose, it rescues the liver by boosting levels of glutathione.

This same effect—glutathione boosting—is also critical for the immune system, especially during times of illness. By increasing glutathione levels, NAC can protect against the excessive free radical activity that comes with being sick.

Since the 1960s, doctors have used an NAC inhalant to treat cystic fibrosis, a disease characterized by the formation of unusually thick mucus that severely hampers normal respiratory function. Scientifically speaking, NAC is a mucolytic agent: It thins out excess mucus by breaking up the sulphur bonds that "glue" mucus together. Less severe and more common medical conditions also involve excess mucus production, including allergies, bad colds, bronchitis, and sinus infections. NAC is effective for those problems as well. I have used NAC (alone or in combination with other immunotics or drugs) to relieve symptoms for my patients with many different types of respiratory problems.

NAC may be of particular value for people with chronic sinusitis, which is fast becoming an epidemic. I see more and more chronic sinus infections that do not respond to standard antibiotic therapy. The warm, moist sinus passages are a wonderful breeding ground for bacteria and fungi, and once the infection sets in, it doesn't want to leave. I often treat people who have taken multiple courses of different antibiotics to no avail. They come to me because they have been told that sinus surgery is their only option. While surgery is supposed to remove the infected tissue and open up the sinuses, it often interferes with the normal sinus mechanism. In the long run, I think it often does more harm than good.

Many postsurgery patients continue to be plagued with chronic sinus infections! My approach is different; I recommend taking 1500 mg of NAC at the *earliest* stage of a sinus infection. It can vastly improve the odds of recovery. People with chronic sinusitis need to take a higher dose. (For more details, see page 177.)

NAC offers wonderful protection against the flu. Older people, in particular, are especially vulnerable to severe, life-threatening bouts of flu. Doctors urge people over age sixty to get annual flu shots, and I wholeheartedly agree. However, while flu shots are great, they don't always work. It's important to have a game plan if the flu should strike—especially for older people. In a placebo-controlled study, physicians at the Institute of Hygiene and Preventive Medicine at the University of Genoa examined the effect of NAC on 262 predominantly older patients who suffered from nonrespiratory chronic ailments for six months. None of the patients received flu vaccinations that year. Patients detailed any flulike symptoms they contracted during the study period on a personal diary card. Every month, researchers evaluated the cards and examined the patients.

The results were quite remarkable. Of the 99 flulike episodes reported in the placebo group, 48 percent were classified as mild, 47 percent as moderate, and 6 percent as severe. Of the 46 flulike episodes reported in the NAC group, 72 percent were classified as mild, 26 percent as moderate, and only 2 percent as severe. Only 9 percent of the patients on NAC, about the same amount who were on the placebo, reported any untoward side effects. When reporting the results of their study in the *European Respiratory Journal,* researchers noted:

NAC treatment was well tolerated and resulted in a significant decrease in the frequency of influenza-like episodes, severity, and length of time confined to bed. . . . Our study shows that the use of a highly tolerable drug such as N-acetyl-cysteine during the cold season is especially advisable in elderly people and high risk individuals.

Everyone should use this immunotic for prevention and treatment of flus in particular and respiratory infections in general. I take it myself!

NAC has other applications as well. I recommend it for my patients with chronic hepatitis C, a terrible virus that slowly destroys the liver and puts sufferers at increased risk of liver cancer. For these patients, NAC serves a dual role. It turns up the immune system, enabling the body to better fight off the acute virus. By stimulating NK cell activity, NAC helps prevent liver cancer. Some studies suggest that NAC may help treat immunodeficiency syndromes such as AIDS. AIDS patients have lower than normal levels of antioxidants, especially the key antioxidant glutathione. In fact, some researchers believe that oxidative stress caused by the depletion of antioxidants may accelerate the progression of HIV infection to AIDS. Scientists who have investigated the effect of NAC on HIV patients have found that it can enhance the response of T-cells. Even though the doses were relatively high (up to 8000 mg daily), NAC was well tolerated. (Please note: I am in no way suggesting that NAC can cure AIDS, but it may be a useful tool to help in the fight.)

Smokers, or those who live or work with smokers, should pay attention to NAC—it may help prevent some of the damage inflicted to lungs by cigarette smoke. Cigarette smoke is a toxic brew of free radicals and other chemicals that quickly depletes glutathione stores in the lining of the lung. Although NAC doesn't offer complete protection against cigarette smoke—nothing can—it may reduce injury to lung cells. In one study, rats exposed to cigarette smoke did not develop the expected precancerous changes in DNA of the cells of their lung or trachea. Of course, NAC pales in comparison to the best remedy: STOP SMOKING.

Much more than just an immunotic to take when you are sick, NAC may play a powerful role in the prevention of heart disease and other diseases of aging. It can reduce the levels of homocysteine, a major risk factor for heart disease, Alzheimer's disease, birth defects, and different types of cancer.

### Olive Leaf Extract*

**Rx:** A natural antimicrobial for all manner of acute infections—antibiotic, antiviral, and antifungal. Part of the Immunotics program for people with chronic GI problems and those who live or work in a high-risk environment.

**The Right Amount:** Range: 500–3000 mg daily. Lower dose: take 1 (500 mg) capsule daily. Higher dose: take 2 (500 mg) capsules up to 3 times daily.

Olive leaf extract tops my list as the treatment of choice for acute colds, flus, respiratory problems, and ear infections. Why? It works quickly, effectively, and without the negative side effects of antibiotics. Of course, I willingly prescribe antibiotics to people who need them—I would be foolish not to. Nor am I suggesting that olive leaf extract or any other immunotic can replace antibiotics in serious infections. However, olive leaf extract is a great tool to have. I turn to olive leaf extract when my patients feel so sick that they beg for an antibiotic, even though their condition does not warrant one. Available in tablet and capsule form, olive leaf extract is destined to become a superstar among the immunotic supplements.

I know from personal experience just how well—and how fast—olive leaf extract works. I rarely get sick (which I attribute to my strict adherence to my Immunotics program!) but when I do, it can be nasty. Recently, I developed a case of bronchitis that seemed to come out of nowhere. As I mentioned earlier, as a child I was prone to respiratory infections. Even now, as an adult, when I am unfortunate enough to catch a head or chest cold, the hacking cough lingers sometimes for weeks on end. True to form, this bout of bronchitis leveled me—I had a high fever and felt utterly miserable. Yet within a few days of taking olive leaf extract, I felt better . . . a lot better. Within a week, the symptoms had vanished. This does not surprise me. I have seen olive leaf extract have a similar positive effect on scores of patients and have personally enjoyed its power many times. Olive leaf extract, I believe, is one of the most powerful antibiotics that nature has to offer.

Like that of human beings, a plant's ability to survive in the wild is dependent on whether it can control bacteria, fungi, molds, and viral invaders. Consequently, plants have a built-in natural pharmacy that keeps them healthy— a pharmacy humans have been tapping for thousands of years. Long before the age of antibiotics, herbal healers used plants to treat many common conditions. This legacy lives on in modern medicine. Nearly 50 percent of all pharmaceutical drugs either derive from plant sources or contain chemical imitations of a plant compound.

The olive tree has been a boon to human health for all of our history. Since biblical times, the fruit of the olive tree has been used for both food and medicine. Today olive oil, the backbone of the Mediterranean diet, is touted as a health food. Numerous studies document that people who eat a diet rich in olive oil have a lower risk of heart disease than those who eat a diet high in the saturated fats (like butter) favored in the United States. Although new to us, olive leaf extract has been used in medicine since the early nineteenth century. Tea brewed from olive leaves, an old European folk remedy for a variety of ills, dates back hundreds of years. In the nineteenth century, scientists studying the chemical structure of the olive leaf discovered a phenolic compound called oleuropein (o-lure-o-peen), but that is only one of the leaf's active ingredients. In the 1960s, researchers at a pharmaceutical company in the United States reported that olive leaf extract could inhibit the growth of viruses, fungi, and other troublesome microorganisms. There was even talk of developing olive leaf as a pharmaceutical drug, but that never came to fruition. I have a hunch that pharmaceutical companies were either discouraged by olive leaf being an unpatentable naturally occurring substance or deemed it was not potent enough to be an effective antibiotic (a point I'll address later).

Perhaps because of the growing problem of antibiotic resistance, scientists have taken a closer look at the olive leaf. Here are some of the most important findings:

*Antimicrobial* Olive leaf extract can inhibit the growth of a wide range of troublesome pathogens, including *Escherichia coli* (E. coli), *Klebsiella pneumoniae, Bacillus cereus, Salmonella enteritidis, Staphylococcus auereus, Candida albicans,* various forms of herpes virus, molds, and parasites.

*Antioxidant* Low-density lipoprotein (LDL) delivers cholesterol to the tissues of the body, but when it becomes oxidized, LDL can lead to clogged arteries (atherosclerosis). Studies have shown that olive leaf extract can prevent the oxidation of LDL, which strongly suggests that it has antioxidant activity. Antioxidants are not just good for your heart but, as you may remember, are also essential for immune function.

*Immune booster* When you are sick, immune cells called macrophages spew out tiny amounts of the body's natural immunotic, nitric oxide, to kill invading microorganisms. Animal studies show that oleuropein enhances the production of nitric oxide by macrophages, giving them more ammunition to fight infection.

In my practice, I have observed that olive leaf extract can speed recovery from colds, flus, and other infections. I mentioned earlier that drug companies may have lost interest in olive leaf extract because it was not as potent as other antibiotics—but this apparent weakness may be its greatest strength. Olive leaf is quite effective against the microbes that cause infection, but it spares the "good" disease-fighting bacteria. It definitely works in a kinder, gentler fashion than prescription antibiotics. There will be times when you may need to take something stronger, but when you don't, olive leaf extract is an excellent alternative. Nor have I found any evidence that olive leaf extract can lead to the development of resistant bacteria. No matter how often I prescribe it, it still seems to do the job. Only more time and research will settle this important point.

As with other immunotics, olive leaf extract may possess some startling *side benefits.* Recently, there has been some debate in the scientific community over the true cause of heart disease. Some studies suggest that bacteria such as chlamydia and *Heliobacter pylori,* the main cause of stomach ulcers, may be the real culprits that cause the heart disease cascade. Whatever the outcome of the debate, taking olive leaf extract not only treats your immediate problem but may prevent even more serious ones down the road.

---

### Probiotics *

**Rx:** These "good" bacteria are so important, they are part of my basic immune-strengthening program for everyone.

**The Right Amount:** Take 1–2 capsules daily, or ½–1 teaspoon of L. acidophilus powder mixed in liquid.

---

*Probiotics,* a word derived from Greek that means *for life,* refers to the numerous microorganisms (or friendly bacteria) that bolster our defenses against disease and play a vital role in digestion. Probiotics help manufacture B vitamins such as niacin, folic acid, and biotin, produce natural antibiotic substances that kill bad bacteria (such as salmonella and E. coli), and manufacture lactase, an enzyme essential for the digestion of dairy products. When taken as a supplement, probiotics can lower blood cholesterol levels.

For two decades, I have prescribed probiotics to my patients, and I'm sure they can benefit just about everyone, especially people who are taking antibiotics or have chronic gut problems, traveler's diarrhea, eczema, chronic fatigue syndrome, or chronic yeast infections.

Friendly bacteria line the intestinal tract, an often overlooked component of the immune system. Everything that passes through your mouth ends up there, and every day the GI tract gets bombarded with chemicals, foreign proteins, free radicals, bacteria, and other organisms that must not enter the bloodstream. It's a demanding job, and that's why 60 percent of the body's immune cells reside in the lining of the gut.

Billions of bacteria live in the GI tract—in fact, there may be more bacteria in the gut than there are cells in the human body! Not all gut bacteria are good; some, like E. coli, are downright harmful. But the primary job of good bacteria in the gut is to inhibit the proliferation of bad bacteria and other harmful pathogens such as fungi. Our health depends on striking the right balance between good and bad bacteria, but unfortunately our modern lifestyle and diet has tipped the odds against us.

The overuse of antibiotics, combined with poor diet, has created potentially harmful changes in the intestinal balance of power. An antibiotic doesn't just kill bad bacteria; it kills the good ones as well. Even if you don't consume antibiotics directly, you may be getting them in food. Over half of the 35 million pounds of antibiotics produced in the United States each year are fed to the livestock from which we get our meat and dairy products, to increase yield and treat infection. Undoubtedly we get some antibiotic residues with each bite of hamburger or glass of milk. To compound the problem, many of us consume diets that are not supportive of friendly bacteria. Good bacteria "eat" dietary fiber and metabolize it into organic acids that inhibit the growth of bad bacteria. Many of us eat fiber-poor diets, unfortunately, resulting in a deficiency of good bacteria and an overgrowth of bad ones.

The intestinal tract harbors hundreds of different species of bacteria, but the most important ones are the lactobacillus and bifidobacteria families. Lactobacilli live in the small and large intestines, while bifidobacteria live only in the large intestine. In infants, bifidobacteria are the primary friendly bacteria, but the balance switches in adulthood. When recommending probiotics, I generally give lactobacillus to adults and bifidobacteria to infants and children under the age of two. If, however, there is evidence of a bifidobacteria deficiency in adults (which can be measured in a stool sample) I will also recommend a bifidobacteria supplement.

Probiotics have a direct impact on immune function. Various studies show that probiotics can boost the level of white blood cells, stimulate phagocytosis (macrophage activity), and increase the production of the immune system's natural antibiotic, gamma-interferon. Some studies have even shown that probiotics can inhibit the growth of cancerous tumors in animals.

Yogurt, the major food source of probiotics (advertised as active cultures on the label) is not necessarily the best source. Many of the live organisms in yogurt get broken down before they can do any good. Therefore, I recommend supplementation as a more efficient way to get your probiotics. (Don't stop eating yogurt—it's still a good food, and I eat it every day!) A final word: one way to avoid getting an extra antibiotic dose with every meal is to eat antibiotic-free milk, poultry, and meat whenever possible.

### St. John's Wort

**Rx:** For people under excessive emotional stress or those suffering mild depression.

**The Right Amount:** Take 1 (300 mg) capsule 3 times daily.

**Special Instructions:** Look for a standardized extract containing 0.3% hypercin with 4–5 hyperforin.

Best known as an over-the-counter treatment for depression, St. John's wort (*Hypericum perforatum*) is often overlooked as a powerful antiviral and antibacterial agent. It is the perfect immunotic for someone under severe stress or suffering from minor depression. As noted earlier, chronic stress significantly dampens immune function and increases the odds of getting sick. When faced with this situation, I like St. John's wort because it not only boosts mood but also gives the immune system much-needed help when necessary. A 1996 study published in the *British Journal of Medicine* reviewed 23 clinical trials involving St. John's wort and concluded that it worked better than a placebo in treating mild to moderate depression. In Germany, where there is a greater acceptance of herbal medicines than in the United States, St. John's wort is the leading antidepressant. Similar to prescription drugs like Prozac, Zoloft, and Paxil, St. John's wort enhances serotonin activity in the brain. Serotonin helps regulate mood, appetite, and sleep, and an imbalance in its levels can trigger mood disorders.

St. John's wort has also been used (along with other conventional therapies) as a treatment for AIDS. Hypericin, an ingredient in St. John's wort, can inhibit the spread of HIV and may also inactivate the virus; at least it has in test tube studies. It also has antibacterial activity. If you have been diagnosed HIV, do not use St. John's wort without your doctor's supervision. Recent studies suggest that St. John's wort may interfere with the efficacy of some antiviral medications used to treat AIDS.

Herbalists have used St. John's wort topically as a treatment for burns and skin irritations, and studies show it can accelerate the healing time for second and third degree burns.

### Siberian Ginseng*

**Rx:** To treat athletes under stress and an aging immune system.

**The Right Amount:** Take 1 (500 mg) capsule twice daily.

Siberian ginseng (Eleutherococcus) is not actually true ginseng (known as Asian, or panax, ginseng); rather, it is a cousin to ginseng, an essential part of Chinese medicine for more than four thousand years. Traditionally, Siberian ginseng is renowned for its ability to both increase athletic endurance and stimulate the immune system. In Western medicine, Siberian ginseng was examined by Soviet scientist

I. I. Brekhman, who in 1969 reported that soldiers who took ginseng extract ran faster in a 3 kilometer race than those taking a placebo. Dr. Brekhman dubbed Siberian ginseng an adaptogen, which he defined as any substance that enables the body to better cope with stress. That is precisely why I recommend Siberian ginseng to my patients who engage in high-level sports or athletic competition. Intense physical activity places the entire body under stress but exacts a particularly steep toll on the immune system. After a rigorous workout, levels of glutathione plummet, a prime reason why marathon runners are vulnerable to respiratory infections after a marathon. The problem is compounded by a sharp rise in cortisol, the stress hormone that dampens immune function and wears athletes down—physically and mentally.

Siberian ginseng enables people to better withstand physical and emotional stress. According to a major study that reviewed clinical trials involving more than two thousand people, Siberian ginseng improves athletic performance, enhances the ability to cope with unpleasant situations (such as excess noise, heat, and high workload), and improves mental alertness. Although its mode of action is not fully understood, some scientists suspect that Siberian ginseng may help reduce stress and enhance well-being by improving the balance among neurotransmitters in the brain. In addition, Siberian ginseng increases T-cells and boosts NK cell activity.

I also recommend Siberian ginseng to people showing signs of immunosenescence. It not only gives their immune system a much-needed boost but increases energy and stamina.

Although Siberian ginseng has many of the same properties as Asian ginseng, there are some important differences.

For one thing, they have different active chemical ingredients. In addition, many people find panax ginseng too stimulating. In some cases, it may cause high blood pressure or insomnia. Siberian ginseng, on the other hand, does not cause jitteriness. It has even been used as a treatment for insomnia.

### Thymic Protein*

**Rx:**  First aid for an aging immune system.

**The Right Amount:**  Thymic protein is an additional immunotic for people following the immunosenescence program. I recommend 1 packet of thymic protein daily (dissolved under the tongue) or up to 3 packets daily in times of increased stress.

The risk of developing cancer or contracting a serious infection rises exponentially as we enter our sixth and seventh decades. Why? Many experts attribute it to a slowdown in immune function. This slowdown has many causes: the age-related reduction in key hormones and the proliferation of free radicals are both likely suspects, but they are not the only cause of immunosenescence. The real answer could be located right under your nose—or more precisely, in the small gland located behind your breastbone called the thymus. As you may remember from chapter 2, the thymus is a pinkish-gray gland that programs T-cells to differentiate between the cells of the body and foreign protein. Starting right after puberty, the thymus begins to shrink and continues to disintegrate until it is entirely replaced by fatty tissue. By age 40, the thymus gland has shrunk to one-sixth of its original size, and in many people is barely discernible. As thymic function decreases, our immune system loses some of its punch.

Until the 1960s, the thymus was considered to be a completely useless gland. (An enlarged thymus was considered a threat to health!) Groundbreaking animal studies showed quite the contrary. Removing the thymus from a young animal not only seriously compromises immune function but also promotes premature aging and early death. Further studies showed that the thymus itself produces hormones that stimulate immune function. But by midlife, we no longer have the benefit of this powerful immunoenhancer.

I recommend that older people (50 and up) take supplemental thymic protein as a way of restoring lost thymic function. Several studies have shown that supplemental thymic protein can, among other things, raise the total number of white blood cells, boost NK cell activity, and increase the level of key T-cells. In human studies, thymic protein helped to suppress flu virus. Anecdotal reports suggest that thymic protein may be useful in treating Epstein-Barr virus, shingles, and hepatitis infections. Yet I think that the real benefit of thymic protein may be in its ability to give a sluggish immune system a much-needed boost so that it can help prevent these infections in the first place.

### Tea Tree Oil*

**Rx:** For skin infections.

**The Right Amount:** Apply directly to infected area up to 4 times daily. (Use 10 percent strength tea tree oil.)

European settlers in Australia learned about tea tree oil (*Melaleuca alternifolia*) from the Aborigines, who used it to treat cuts, wounds, and fungal infections. Despite its name, tea tree oil is not derived from the tea plant from which we get the famous beverage. Its name stems from the Aboriginal practice of making a tea from it to use in healing.

Tea tree is an excellent antiseptic with natural antibacterial and antifungal properties as well. I recommend it for external use only, primarily for my patients with athlete's foot or toenail fungus. If you have sensitive skin, however, do not use tea tree oil. Please be careful: I have seen tea tree oil cause severe allergic reactions in some people, notably those with a tendency to get skin rashes.

### Uva Ursi*

**Rx:** For urinary tract and bladder infections.

**The Right Amount:** Take 1 dropperful of tincture 4 times daily.

Uva ursi (*Arctostaphylos uva ursi*) is a small evergreen plant that has been used as a natural diuretic and antiseptic in folk medicine for many centuries. I prescribe this herb to patients with mild urinary tract infections who do not have fever, back pain, nausea, or any other signs that the infection has spread. (If you have signs of a serious infection, you *must* take a stronger prescription antibiotic.) Many urinary tract infections are growing resistant to antibiotics, resulting in patients having to take several different courses of antibiotics to beat the bug. Rather than going through that, I try uva ursi first whenever possible. It often stops the infection in its earliest stages and, although it is a natural antibiotic, does not appear to create resistant strains. Uva ursi works best in a nonacidic environment; therefore, do not take this herb with vitamin C or orange juice. You need not avoid acidic foods and supplements all day, but do wait a few minutes after taking uva ursi.

---

**Western Larch\***
**Rx:** Good for colds, ear infections, and flu.
**The Right Amount:** Take ½ teaspoon powder mixed in liquid 3 times daily.

---

The western larch tree *(Larix occidentalis)* is ubiquitous throughout the western United States. Western larch contains a type of polysaccharide called arabinogalactan and is similar in chemical structure to some other immunotics (echinacea, astragalus, and shiitake). Larch extract, refined into a cream-colored powder, is my treatment of choice for children with colds, ear infections, and flus. Those conditions, for which there are few conventional treatments, leave children (and parents!) miserable. For them, larch is a wonder drug. Both easy to use and very effective, larch frees children from having to swallow pills or drink icky-tasting extract (the powder is mixed with a small amount of warm water and then diluted in a glass of juice.) Fairly inexpensive, larch is also very safe—so safe that it has been approved by the FDA as a stabilizer and thickening agent for powdered puddings.

I have seen larch work wonders, especially for the children who get cold after cold or who have been on a string of antibiotics, and can't seem to get well. Larch gives the child's immune system an edge, helping him or her shake off the infection for good.

The Max Planck Institute in Germany studied larch and found that it can boost NK cell activity. It also has natural antiviral activity: While the revitalized NK cells are seeking and destroying the viral invaders, larch assists in the destruction.

The good news about larch is that it is an excellent source of fiber, but the bad news is that fiber may cause a gassy stomach. However, the discomfort is rarely serious, especially for those people who are used to high-fiber diets. Given all the good things larch does, I highly recommend it, despite this minor problem.

Larch is not just for children. Like olive leaf extract, larch is a great immunotic to turn to when fighting a cold or flu. It's especially good for people who are looking for an alternative to echinacea. As I said earlier, I do not believe that you should rely on one immunotic alone. With larch, echinacea, and olive leaf extract, colds and flus don't have a chance!

# FIVE

# The Immunotics Program

**Y**ou have now learned about the importance of the immune system, seen how it works, and discovered the powerful effect immunotics can have. Now it's time to make the Immunotics program work for you.

When you strengthen your immune system, you don't just aid one system in your body. All the good things that you are doing for your immune system will benefit every other system, from your brain to your heart. The effects of the Immunotics program are palpable. You will feel better. You will look better. You will have better resistance against disease. If you do get sick, your body will heal faster.

In order to reap the full benefit of Immunotics, however,

you need to tune into the four separate but essential components of this program. Each part of the Immunotics program
is powerful on its own, but combined they are especially potent against the forces of disease.

## I. Your Personal Immunotics Prescription

Chapter 4, "The Immunotics Pharmacy," reviews the 30 different immunotic supplements, illustrating their dosage, indication, and use. In chapter 6, "Your Personal Immunotics
Prescription," we will pull all of this information together
and outline which immunotics you should take every day
and which ones you should reserve for special situations. We
will also review the health challenges facing many individuals
today, and present a specialized Immunotics plan for each.

> *The basics* First, everyone should follow the basic plan,
> listed on pages 150–51. It is a simple but highly effec-
> tive program for general immune support. Everyone
> who breathes should follow the basic plan. It provides
> immune enhancement for everyone! For those with
> specific challenges, there are nine other specialized
> plans designed to meet their needs. Some of you will
> immediately know which plan applies to you, while oth-
> ers may need to refer back to chapter 3 to determine if
> you have any risk factors that warrant additional im-
> mune support.
>
> *Aging* Plan 2 is geared to people aged 50 or older who
> need extra immune support.
>
> *High risk* Plan 3 helps people living or working in high-
> risk environments—such as hospital workers, parents

of young children, school teachers, and people working in poorly ventilated offices.

*Stress* Plan 4 controls the negative effects of excessive emotional stress.

*Cancer* Plan 5 is for people who are at high risk of developing cancer, based on family medical history and lifestyle.

*GI problems* Plan 6 is for people who fall prey to common gastrointestinal problems such as irritable bowel, ulcers, indigestion, and stomach "flu."

*Respiratory ailments* Plan 7 helps people who have chronic respiratory infections, sinus infections, or allergies.

*Athletes* Plan 8 keeps endurance athletes healthy—even after a vigorous workout, when they are most vulnerable to infection.

*Travelers* Plan 9 is for travelers, especially those going to countries that have questionable water quality and sanitation.

*Children* Plan 10 supports children who are getting cold after cold, virus after virus, and can't seem to get well.

Depending on your particular circumstance, you may follow different programs at different times. For example, if you are generally well but are planning to travel to a Third World country, you may need to follow the travelers program for the duration of your trip. If you are a parent of a child who gets sick frequently in the winter, you might consider switching to the high-risk program for yourself during cold and flu season. Or, if you have severe allergies, you may want to follow the program for respiratory ailments during allergy season.

As good as this supplement regimen is—and believe me, I've seen it work wonders—it cannot do the job alone. You still need to follow the second part of the Immunotics program, the Immunotics food plan.

## II. How to Feed Your Immune System

Immune system enemy number one isn't anything you've heard about yet—not some deadly virus or killer bacteria. It's what we are putting on our plates. Believe it or not, poor nutrition is the leading cause of weakened immune function. We eat too much of the wrong foods and too little of the right ones. Not only is that a recipe for illness, it is also the major reason why one out of four American adults is clinically obese.

A good diet is the best immunotic. In chapter 8, I outline exactly what you need to eat to strengthen your immune system and improve your overall health. I'm not asking you to make radical changes in your diet, nor would I advocate anything weird or trendy that you could never follow for more than a few weeks. Rather, the Immunotics food plan asks you to take stock of what and how you eat and to make some simple changes.

As you will see in chapter 8, it is easier than you think to use the power of food to revitalize your immune system. Specifically, I will show you how to incorporate immune-boosting *superfoods* into your daily diet—foods that are packed with beneficial phytochemicals that fight against disease and fortify the immune system—while alerting you to *immune zappers*.

Adding seven to ten servings of superfoods to your daily diet will make an enormous difference in your overall health and the health of your immune system. At the same time, you'll do yourself a world of good. The foods that support immune function also protect against heart disease, cancer, diabetes, and other common ailments!

## III. Tapping the Power of Your Mind

Your mind—your thoughts and feelings—can be a powerful immunotic, if you know how to use it. Creating the right mental environment is an essential tool in maintaining your health—as important, even, as taking your supplements and eating the right foods. On the other hand, a barrage of negative thoughts and beliefs can hamper the effectiveness of the most powerful Immunotics program.

In chapter 9, I will show you how to use your mind as an immunotic. This chapter is not only geared for those of you who are well and looking to stay that way, but it will benefit people suffering from chronic illness.

## IV. Creating an Immune-friendly Environment

The final component of the Immunotics program encourages you to re-examine your habits and lifestyle. In chapter 10, I will give specific advice on how people with risk factors can reduce their exposure. More important, I will give valuable information on how to prevent problems in the first place—particularly for people in high-risk situations.

In the chapter that follows, select the immunotics supplement regimen that best suits your needs. As powerful as immunotic supplements are, you will not experience their full impact unless you take them every day. Make it as much a part of your daily life as brushing your teeth! In the chapters to come, I will show you how easy it is to incorporate the other equally important aspects of the Immunotics program into your life.

# SIX

# Your Personal Immunotics Prescription

The right combination of supplements can help you maintain a strong, well-functioning immune system. It is a simple and effective way to give your immune system the "fuel" it needs to keep you well. This is the heart of the Immunotics program.

The Basic Immunotics Program can be of benefit to anyone who wants to maintain his or her health now and in later years. But everybody is not the same, and some people have specific concerns. For that reason, I have modified my basic plan to accommodate people with special needs, such as those experiencing the age-related decline in immune function, those under extreme stress, those in high-risk situations, and school-aged children, who are virtual magnets for every bug that comes their way.

All of the immunotics mentioned in this chapter were discussed in further detail in chapter 4, "The Immunotic Pharmacy." If you have any questions about a particular supplement, refer to chapter 4 for an in-depth explanation.

*Where can I buy my immunotic supplements?*

Twenty years ago, when I first began recommending immunotic supplements, my patients had a heck of a time finding them. Today, high-quality supplements can be purchased at natural food stores, pharmacies, discount drugstores, general merchandise stores, supermarkets, and even on the Internet. Incidentally, prices vary widely on supplements, so watch for sales. Some chains offer discounts to frequent supplement buyers or to seniors. Some of the larger chains even have special two-for-one sales on brand-name supplements, which can save quite a bit of money.

*Which brand should I buy?*

It all depends on the immunotic. In many cases, one brand is as good as the next, and you can purchase whichever brand you prefer. In some cases, however, I recommend a specific brand. See the Resources section at the end of the book for a list of the recommended brands. Here are some other tips on how to choose the right brand of supplement:

- Stick to brands produced by reputable, well-known manufacturers who take special steps to ensure safety and effectiveness.
- Look for products that come in sealed, tamper-proof packages with both an inside and outside seal.

○ Always select products that say on the label that they are laboratory tested and guaranteed, which means that the contents have been assayed by an independent laboratory.

○ If possible, buy products with expiration dates, since some herbs and other supplements can lose potency over time.

(Unless the label specifies that you need to refrigerate a product, store your supplement in a cool, dry place out of direct sunlight.)

*What do the dosage numbers mean?*

Immunotics are micronutrients, meaning you need only to ingest a comparatively small amount to get a good result. While immunotics are usually measured in milligrams or grams (as in the case of powders), when I recommend an extract (like grapefruit seed extract or tea tree oil), the dose is in drops. For example, I may tell you to use 10 drops of grapefruit seed extract diluted in water up to 3 times daily. Probiotics are another exception to the rule. They are usually measured in terms of the number of live active cells per capsule.

At times I may recommend taking an additional vitamin or mineral supplement. Vitamins are organic substances essential for life that are found in food. Most vitamins are water soluble (like B vitamins and C)—not stored in body fat; you excrete any excess quantity. Fat-soluble vitamins (such as A and E) are stored by the body; the body does not eliminate excess amounts. Fat-soluble vitamins are measured in international units (IUs), milligrams, or retinol equivalents (REs).

Minerals are naturally occurring chemical elements necessary for body processes such as the formation of strong teeth and bones, muscle movements, and normal cell function. Minerals come in two categories: essential minerals and trace minerals. Essential minerals, which we need more of, as the name implies, are measured in milligrams or grams. Trace minerals are measured in micrograms (one-millionth of a gram.).

*Why do you recommend a dose range
as opposed to a specific dose?*

The amount of supplement required to achieve the right result often varies from person to person. Prescription drugs are similarly variable. To accommodate individual differences, my recommended dose for a particular supplement often allows for flexibility. You know your body best—if you tend to respond strongly to medication, start with the lower dose and work your way up to the higher one, if necessary.

*Are immunotics safe for children?*

**Unless I list an immunotic as safe for children, I do not recommend that you use it on your kids.** This doesn't mean that the immunotic isn't safe, only that I have not had extensive experience using it on children or do not have in-depth research on juvenile use. In the absence of either of those two things, I do not feel comfortable recommending it to others. The immunotics that I recommend for children are only those that I have successfully and safely used in my practice. I caution you against giving children pills or tablets to swallow on which they could choke. For small children especially, use only chewable tablets, liquid extracts, or powders that can be dissolved in water or juice. Do not use any immunotic on a child under six months of age. Children should not follow the Basic Immunotics Program; to accommodate their special needs, I have designed a special program (see page 158).

*Can I take immunotics with other medications?*
In most cases, yes—with some important exceptions. Do not use any immunotic if you have recently undergone an organ transplant and are taking immunosuppressive drugs to prevent the rejection of the organ. (In this situation, your best bet is to avoid exposure to infection as much as possible while your immune defenses are down. For some good tips on staying well, read chapter 10, "Creating an Immune-Friendly Environment.")

There are other situations where medication and immunotics may not mix. I believe it is important for patients to tell their physicians what vitamins, herbs, or other immunotics they take. Some immunotics (such as vitamin E, ginkgo, and garlic) enhance the effects of blood thinners like Coumadin, which in rare cases may cause hemorrhaging.

It is particularly important for you to notify your physician about your supplement regimen if you are scheduled for surgery. Some immunotics may interfere with blood clotting—which is good if you want to prevent heart disease but awful if you bleed excessively during surgery. You may need to discontinue taking your immunotic a week or two before and after your surgery. Talk to your doctor for specific advice.

*When should I take an immunotic supplement to treat a problem, and when should I call my doctor?*
Immunotic supplements are great for conditions that you would normally treat without consulting your doctor—com-

mon colds, mild sore throats, stomach bugs, viral infections, and the like. There are times, however, when you should not attempt to treat your own problem. **If you are running a high fever for more than 24 hours, are vomiting excessively, are dizzy, have chest pains, or are feeling very sick, call your physician!** In these situations, do not attempt to self-medicate with either an immunotic or an antibiotic. Your doctor should make the judgment call as to whether you need to be seen. Even if you are sick enough to see a doctor, it doesn't necessarily mean that an antibiotic is in order. Keep in mind that you could have a severe viral infection such as the flu. In this situation, the right immunotic can help speed recovery and get you back on your feet faster, while an antibiotic will do exactly nothing.

*When should I take my supplements?*

I usually recommend that you take your supplements with meals to enhance absorption and prevent stomach upset. In some cases, however, I will tell you to take a specific supplement on an empty stomach. In that case, you should take it either two hours after or one hour before a meal. I personally take my supplements with breakfast and dinner because that's the most convenient for me. If you can't bear the thought of breakfast, plan on taking your supplements with lunch or dinner. This may require that you carry a bag of supplements with you when you go out during the day or leave a set of supplements at the office. If you eat on the run, make it easy on yourself: Take five minutes over the weekend to pack up your week's supply of supplements in small bags so that they are ready when you leave the house in the morning. Whatever you do, be sure to take your supplements consistently, or you will not experience the full benefits of the Immunotics program.

If you are suffering from an acute illness (like a bad cold or stomach virus) you may need to take your supplements more frequently. For more information, see chapter 7.

*Which forms of supplements are the most effective?*
Immunotic supplements are sold in many different forms, from pills to capsules to powders to extracts to teas. Depending on the supplement, the form in which you take it may influence how well it is absorbed by the body. I will tell you which form I think is best. When it comes to children, powders and nonalcoholic extracts are the best because many children simply can't or won't swallow pills, and alcohol and kids don't mix. The same may be true for older people who have difficulty swallowing pills or who need to avoid alcohol. You can mix bitter or bad-tasting immunotics with juice to mask the flavor.

*Can I overdose on immunotic supplements?*
The immunotic supplements listed in this book are nontoxic even at high doses. That doesn't mean that if you take an excessive amount you won't suffer any consequences. In high doses, some immunotics cause stomach upset, diarrhea, and insomnia. To be on the safe side, stick to my recommended doses—you won't run into any trouble!

*What are the new labels for supplements?*
The FDA has recently issued new labeling requirements for dietary supplements. Nutritional supplements—all herbs, vitamins, minerals, and amino acids—must now have a "Supplement Facts" label similar to the "Nutrition Facts" panel on

food labels. These new labels detail the quantity of the main supplement or supplements included in the product in addition to the complete list of other ingredients. In the case of herbs, manufacturers have to specify what part of the plant (root, leaf, or stem) the product derives from.

*Can I also take a multivitamin?*
Sure. Taking a multivitamin along with the Immunotics program is a good combination. In some cases your multivitamin may include some of the immunotics already in your plan; in that case, consider yourself covered—you don't need to take an additional amount. In many cases, however, the multivitamin may not have enough, in which case take enough to get yourself up to the right amount.

## The Immunotics Program for Everybody: The Basic Program

Designed for people who do not have specific risk factors, the Basic Immunotics Program offers general immune support. The basic program includes four key immunotics: a combination antioxidant, a bioflavonoid, a probiotic, and colostrum. Take these immunotics daily.

### Antioxidants

There are numerous antioxidant products on the market that conform to my recommendations, but you may have to take more than one capsule a day. As explained earlier, water-soluble antioxidants pass through the system quickly, so instead of taking the entire dose at once, divide the dose in half. Take the first half in the morning and the second half later in the day. Chewable antioxidants are available for children. Look for an antioxidant complex that includes the following:

| | |
|---|---|
| *Carotenoids:* | A complete complex including 15,000–20,000 mg of beta carotene along with alpha carotene, lutein, and lycopene. |
| *Vitamin E:* | 400 IU of mixed tocopherols, including gamma tocopherol. |
| *Zinc chelate:* | 25–50 mg. |
| *Selenium:* | 100–200 mcg. |
| *Vitamin C:* | 1000–2000 mg. |

**Bioflavonoids**

You can take either of the following:

| | |
|---|---|
| Mixed citrus bioflavonoids: | 1000–1500 mg. |
| Proanthocyanadins (PCOs): | 75–150 mg. |

**Probiotics**

You can take either of the following:

| | |
|---|---|
| *Lactobacillus GG:* | Take 1 capsule. |
| *L-acidophilus:* | Take 1 teaspoon of powder daily. |

| | |
|---|---|
| **Colostrum** | Take 2 (480 mg) capsules on an empty stomach. |

## Immunotics for Special Needs

As I explained in chapter 3, many of us have risk factors in our lives that can have an adverse effect on immune function. Age, exposure to infection, living or working in a toxic environment, and even excessive stress can all depress immunity. Fortunately, you don't have to take it lying down—there is a solution! In addition to following the Basic Immunotics Program, you need to take additional immunotics.

The nine additional programs that follow are tailored to meet specific needs. They will help overcome your risk factors and reclaim—and keep—your health. **These special programs are meant to be followed** *in addition* **to the Basic Immunotics Program.**

For People with an Aging Immune System

If you are over 50 and find that you don't have the resistance that you used to have or can't bounce back as fast from common ailments as you once did, this program can help revive your flagging immune system. In addition to the basic program, take the following immunotics daily.

| | |
|---|---|
| *Alkylglycerol:* | Take 500 mg. |
| *Zinc chelate:* | Take an additional 25 mg for a maximum of 75 mg. |
| *Colostrum:* | Take an additional 4 capsules on an empty stomach (for a total of 6). |
| *CoQ-10:* | Take 100 mg. |
| *Siberian Ginseng:* | Take 500 mg. |

**Optional:** Add these supplements to your regimen if you are experiencing a significant decline in immune function:

| | |
|---|---|
| *7 KETO DHEA:* | Take 25–50 mg, depending on your blood test (see section on 7 KETO DHEA in chapter 4). |
| *Thymic protein:* | Take 1–2 packets daily. |

## For People Working or Living in a High-Risk Environment

If you are a school teacher, a hospital worker, or the parent of a school-aged child and find that you are constantly getting sick, it's time to bring out the big guns. This program will give you the added ammunition you need to keep infection at bay. It won't make you invincible to illness (you still need to eat well, get enough sleep, and follow the advice listed in chapter 9) but you'll feel that way! In addition to the basic program, take the following immunotics daily.

| | |
|---|---|
| *Astragalus:* | Take 500 mg. |
| *Alkylglycerol:* | Take 500 mg. |
| *Olive leaf extract:* | Take 500 mg. |
| *Colostrum:* | Take an additional 4 capsules on an empty stomach. |
| *Garlic:* | Take 900 mg. |
| *Shiitake mushroom:* | Take 500 mg. |

## For People under Extreme Emotional Stress

Intense and prolonged stress can throw your immune system out of balance, leaving you vulnerable to illness and out of kilter. An extremely stressful situation requires you to do more than normal to simply maintain immune function. You must help your body and mind cope with the situations causing upset. Be vigilant about eating well and getting enough rest. Don't push yourself to the limit when you are stressed out—give yourself time to recover. Those last two sentences might contain the most potent immunotics of all! The goal of the program listed here is to bolster immune function while mitigating the negative physical side effects of stress. In addition to the basic program, take the following immunotics daily.

| | |
|---|---|
| *Siberian ginseng:* | Take 500 mg. |
| *Reishi mushroom:* | Take 1000 mg. |
| *St. John's wort:* | Take 900 mg. |

### For People at Higher Risk of Cancer

If you have a strong family history of cancer (defined as having a close relative who died of cancer before age 60), you may be at a greater risk of developing cancer yourself. However, when it comes to assessing cancer risk, genetics is not the only concern. Your cancer risk is also higher if you smoke, have a history of drug or alcohol abuse, or are exposed to carcinogens on the job. If you do face a greater risk of developing cancer, *you must* keep your immune system strong. I recommend the following immunotics daily, in addition to the basic program.

| | |
|---|---|
| *Maitake mushroom:* | Take 1 dropperful. |
| *D-Fraction:* | |
| *Alkylglycerol:* | Take 1000 mg. |

| | |
|---|---|
| *Garlic:* | Take 600 mg dried garlic. |
| *IP-6:* | Take 3–4 capsules. |
| *MGN-3:* | Take 1000 mg. |
| *Astragalus:* | Take 1000 mg. |
| *Green tea extract:* | Take 500 mg. |
| *Curcumin:* | Take 500 mg. |

## For People with Chronic GI Problems

Here comes help for this often overlooked but critical component of the immune system. Suffering from chronic GI problems—indigestion, irritable bowel, ulcers, or reflux disease—not only interferes with your quality of life but also makes you more vulnerable to other nasty ailments, or even cancer. And, as those of you with chronic gut problems already know, it feels like you're a magnet for every stomach bug or flu. Therefore, I urge you to take steps to heal your gut while fortifying your immune system. My immunotics program for chronic gut problems does both, safely and gently. In addition to the basic program, take the following immunotics daily.

| | |
|---|---|
| *L-glutamine:* | Take 1–2 teaspoons in liquid. |
| *Colostrum:* | Take an additional 4 capsules on an empty stomach. |
| *Quercetin:* | Take 2000 mg. |
| *Garlic:* | Take 900 mg dried garlic. |
| *Olive leaf:* | Take 1000 mg. |
| *Aloe vera:* | Take ½ teaspoon in liquid. |
| *(freeze-dried gel)* | |

For People with Chronic Respiratory Problems

Does every cold go into your chest? Do you suffer from frequent sinus problems? Is your respiratory system your Achilles heel? My Immunotics program for people with chronic respiratory problems serves two purposes: it helps to strengthen your respiratory system while giving it the extra boost it needs to ward off infections. Some people may need to follow this program year round if they suffer from respiratory ailments regardless of the season. Others may need it only during times that they are most vulnerable to respiratory problems, such as the flu or allergy season. In addition to the basic program, take the following immunotics as needed.

| | |
|---|---|
| *NAC:* | Take 2000 mg. |
| *Quercetin:* | Take 3000 mg. |
| *Garlic:* | Take 900 mg dried garlic. |
| *Astragalus:* | Take 1500 mg. |
| *Olive leaf:* | Take 1500 mg. |

For Endurance Athletes

You run the marathon, and then what happens? You get knocked off your (sore) feet with a severe upper respiratory infection! Exercise is a good thing, but heavy training and intense physical activity can weaken your immune system. If you engage in vigorous workouts, are training for a special event such as a marathon, or are a competitive athlete, you need some special immunotics help. In addition to the basic program, take the following immunotics daily.

| | |
|---|---|
| *L-glutamine:* | Take 5000 mg on an empty stomach before you work out, and 5000 mg after your workout. |
| *Colostrum:* | Take 4 *additional* capsules daily on an empty stomach (for a total of 6). |
| *NAC:* | Take 2000 mg. |
| *Siberian ginseng:* | Take 1000 mg. |
| *Reishi mushroom:* | Take 1000 mg. |
| *Proanthocyanidins:* *(PCOs)* | Take an additional 300 mg. |
| *CoQ-10:* *(antioxidant)* | Take 100 mg. |
| *Lipoic acid:* *(antioxidant)* | Take 100 mg. |

For Travelers

Travel can be exciting and rewarding, but when you're on the road, you're eating different food, drinking different water, and, most important, getting exposed to different germs. You need to fortify yourself so that you don't ruin your trip by getting sick or come back wrung out instead of well rested. While traveling, in addition to the basic program, take the following immunotics daily.

| | |
|---|---|
| *Probiotics* | |
| *Lactobacillus GG:* | Take 1 *additional* capsule. |
| *or* | |
| *L-acidophilus:* | Take 1 *additional* teaspoon of powder. (Look for |

|  |  |
|---|---|
|  | products guaranteed to contain 2.5 billion organisms per gram.) |
| *Berberine:* | Take 600–900 mg. |
| *Grapefruit seed extract:* | Take 15 drops twice daily in 8 ounces of juice. |

### For School-Aged Children

Children are notoriously picky eaters. They'll eat one kind of food to the exclusion of all others. Many scorn fruits and vegetables, and too often we parents let them eat meals on the run. As a result, children are particularly vulnerable to micronutrient deficiency. This further taxes a growing immune system. To compound the problem, children spend a great deal of time in overheated, stuffy classrooms that breed colds and flus as well as any petri dish! My Immunotics program for children is designed to help youngsters overcome these problems. **CHILDREN SHOULD NOT FOLLOW THE BASIC PROGRAM: THEY SHOULD ONLY TAKE THE FOLLOWING IMMUNOTICS.**

|  |  |
|---|---|
| *Antioxidant complex:* | Take a chewable antioxidant complex designed for children (about ½ adult dose). |
| *Carotenoids:* | A complete complex including 7500 mg beta carotene plus alpha carotene, lutein, and lycopene. |
| *Vitamin E:* | Take 100 IU. |
| *Zinc chelate:* | Take 15 mg. |

| | |
|---|---|
| *Selenium:* | Take 75 mcg. |
| *Vitamin C:* | Take 500 mg. |
| *Astragalus tincture:* | Take 1 dropperful. |
| *Western larch:* | Take ½–1 teaspoon powder mixed in juice. |
| *Flaxseed:* *(fresh ground)* | Take 1 tablespoon in food. |

The Immunotics programs outlined in this chapter are designed to keep you healthy. At times of illness, however, you may need to change your regimen. In the next chapter I show you how to use immunotics to treat common ailments, both acute and chronic.

# SEVEN

# Immunotics for Whatever Ails You

**S**o far we've concentrated on maintaining a strong, well-functioning immune system better able to resist disease, but even the strongest system occasionally fails. You may still suffer from the occasional cold, flu bug, or from a more serious problem. Immunotics can be of even greater value to you then—it is the second half of their promise. Immunotics reduce your chances of getting sick, but if you do fall ill, they'll get you better faster. For many common conditions—from colds to sinus infections to stomach ulcers—immunotics can reduce symptoms, speed up your recovery, and prevent a recurrence.

When you are sick, you need to add immunotics to your

basic daily regimen (see chapter 6) or increase the doses of the immunotics that you are already taking. In the pages that follow, I give you specific information on how much of which immunotics you should take, and for how long, for each problem listed.

**As noted in chapter 6, do not give immunotics (or any other medicine) to infants six months old or younger unless directed by your doctor. Due to their smaller size, children between the ages of three and five should take half the adult dose. After age five, or once a child weighs 60-plus pounds, the adult dose is fine. Do not give small children pills or capsules—they may choke on them.**

Depending on your problem, follow the appropriate program in addition to your basic immunotics regimen. Before you begin, a word of caution. There are times when immunotics can do the job, and there are times when you absolutely must call your doctor—I tell you when those times are. Please follow my advice!

### Respiratory Allergies and Asthma

Respiratory allergies are caused by a hypersensitivity to pollen, dust, animal dander, molds, mites, and/or pollutants in the environment. Severe allergic responses can trigger bronchial asthma, in which the air tubes of the lungs become constricted, making breathing difficult. Antihistamines—either prescription or over the counter—are the usual treatment for respiratory allergies. There are numerous antihistamines, and although they generally work for most people, they are not without side effects. Antihistamines work by stopping a body process—they work against as opposed to with the body. The Immunotics program for allergies aims to relieve the annoying symptoms and gently support immune function.

**Symptoms:** Itchy eyes, nasal congestion, and wheezing.

**Rx:** In addition to the Basic Immunotics Program, take the following supplements:

| | |
|---|---|
| *Quercetin:* | Take 2000–3000 mg daily. |
| *NAC:* | Take 1500–3000 mg daily. |
| *Probiotics:* | Take an additional capsule of Lactobacillus GG daily (for a total of 2 capsules) or an additional teaspoon of L-acidophilus powder daily (for a total of 2 teaspoons.) |
| *Vitamin C:* | Take an additional 1000–2000 mg for a total of 3000 mg daily. |

In addition to these immunotics, I also recommend that allergy sufferers take 300 mg of gamma linolenic acid (GLA). It's not an immunotic, but it is a natural anti-inflammatory and helps to soothe the immune system. The best sources of GLA are borage, evening primrose, and black currant seed oil, which are sold in health food stores.

**WARNING: Call your physician if you experience progressive shortness of breath, fever, or persistent sinus pain or pressure. People with asthma should be under a physician's care and should consult with him or her before taking any medication.**

## Bladder Infections
## (Urinary Tract Infections)

Bladder infections (also known as cystitis) result from the inflammation of the urinary tract, most commonly caused by E. coli bacteria. In severe or persistent infection, antibiotics may be necessary. Due to anatomical differences, women are *25 times* more vulnerable to bladder infections than men!

**Symptoms:** Urgent need to urinate, frequent urination, burning with urination.

**Rx:** In addition to the Basic Immunotics Program, take the following supplements for 3–5 days:

| | |
|---|---|
| *Cranberry extract:* | Take 2 capsules as a "loading dose" and then 1 capsule every 3 hours for up to 6 capsules daily. After the first day, take 1 capsule every 4–6 hours for a total of up to 6 capsules. |
| *Uva ursi:* | Take 1 dropperful of tincture every 3–4 hours. |
| *Probiotics:* | Take an additional capsule of Lactobacillus GG (for a total of 2 capsules)or an additional teaspoon of powder (for a total of 2 teaspoons) daily . |

During the acute phase of the infection, drink at least 1 glass of water every waking hour.

**WARNING: Call your physician immediately if symptoms persist for more than 3 days or if you experience fever, blood in the urine, back pain (especially in the low back around the kidneys), nausea, or vomiting, all of which could indicate that the infection has spread to the kidneys. IF YOU ARE PREGNANT, DO NOT SELF-MEDICATE! At the first sign of a bladder infection, call your doctor.**

## Bronchitis

Bronchitis is inflammation of the lining of the bronchial tubes, often caused by an upper respiratory viral infection. When a cold "goes into your chest," you're feeling a case of bronchitis coming on. Antibiotics don't help, but immunotics can!

**Symptoms:** Annoying, hacking cough, either dry or accompanied by clear mucus, low-grade fever (up to 102 degrees), and mild chest discomfort with deep inhalation.

**Rx:** In addition to the Basic Immunotics Program, take the following supplements for 1–2 weeks. Symptoms should lessen within 3–5 days.

| | |
|---|---|
| *Olive leaf extract:* | Take 2000–3000 mg daily. |
| *Garlic:* | Take 900 mg daily. |
| *NAC:* | Take 3000 mg daily. |
| *Echinacea:* | Take 1 dropperful every 2–3 hours or up to 2 (500 mg) capsules every 4–5 hours. |
| *Citrus bioflavonoids:* | Take an additional |

|  | 1500 mg for a total of 3000 mg daily. |
|---|---|
| *Vitamin C:* | Take an additional 3000–4000 mg daily for a total of 5000 mg daily. (Take the full dose if you can tolerate it, but if you get an upset stomach or diarrhea, cut back to a less irritating dose.) |

**WARNING: Call your physician if you experience short-ness of breath (especially at rest) or rapid breathing, develop a fever of over 102 degrees, or cough up thick, yellow or green mucus or blood.**

### Cancer Support

Cancer should only be diagnosed and treated by a competent medical professional. Immunotics can support conventional cancer treatment but cannot substitute for state-of-the-art cancer therapies! Immunotics can help conventional therapies work better, but to rely on them alone puts your life at risk. Please find an open-minded physician who will work closely with you to design the right cancer treatment program for you. If you are under treatment for cancer, check all medications and supplements with your physician before taking them.

**Rx:** Depending on the particular cancer, I often recommend some or all of these immunotics to my cancer patients who need general immune boosting. These supplements can be taken indefinitely, but lower doses may be used during times of remission. Please consult with your physician before beginning.

| | |
|---|---|
| *MGN-3:* | Take 2000–3000 mg daily. |
| *IP-6:* | Take 9–12 capsules daily. |
| *Alkylglycerol:* | Take 1500 mg daily. |
| *Garlic:* | Take 900 mg daily. |
| *NAC:* | Take 3000 mg daily. |
| *Astragalus:* | Take 1500 mg daily. |
| *Vitamin C:* | Take 3000–5000 mg daily up to GI tolerance. |
| *OPC:* | Take 300 mg daily. |
| *CoQ-10:* | Take 200–400 mg daily. |
| *Curcumin:* | Take 1000–1500 mg daily. |
| *Green tea extract:* | Take 1000 mg daily. |

**WARNING: If you are undergoing chemotherapy, alert your oncologist that you are taking immunotics. Do not use immunotics if you are taking an immunosuppressant drug, as in the case of people undergoing bone marrow transplants.**

## Colds (Upper Respiratory Infections)

Caused by the rhinovirus family, the cold is the single most common ailment affecting humans! The average adult suffers through two to three colds a year, while the average school-aged child endures up to six colds a year. What we lump together as the common cold may be caused by more than one hundred different viruses. The cure for the common cold still eludes us, but immunotics can reduce the severity of symptoms and speed recovery.

**Symptoms:**  Sinus congestion, runny nose, sore throat, swollen glands in neck, cough, low-grade fever (under 102 degrees). You generally feel miserable!

**Rx:**  Take these supplements for 7–14 days, depending on how fast you recover.

| | |
|---|---|
| *Echinacea:* | Take 1 dropperful every 2–3 hours or up to 2 (500 mg) capsules every 4–5 hours. |
| *Astragalus:* | Take 1 dropperful of tincture every 2–3 hours or capsules equivalent to 1500 mg daily. |
| *Garlic:* | Take 900 mg daily. |
| *Olive leaf extract:* | Take 2000–3000 mg daily. |
| *Citrus bioflavonoids:* | Take an additional 1500 mg for a total of 3000 mg daily. |
| *Vitamin C:* | Take an additional 1000–2000 mg for a total of 3000 mg daily. |

**WARNING: Call your physician if you experience shortness of breath (especially at rest), rapid breathing, or fever of over 102 degrees, or if you cough up thick, yellow or green mucus or blood.**

## Cold Sores and Blisters

Cold sores are fever blisters, usually on or around the mouth, caused by the herpes simplex type I virus. Its more famous sibling, herpes simplex type II, causes herpes in the genital area and sometimes on other parts of the body. Either form is painful. Herpes is one of the most common of all infections. About 90 percent of the U. S. population has had some form of herpes virus; an astonishing fifty million people have had genital herpes. Cold sores are spread through kissing or the use of the same glass or utensils. Genital herpes is passed through sexual contact, but the infected person isn't always aware that he or she is carrying the virus. In fact, herpes simplex II can lie dormant for years and then strike again without notice. Vigilant use of condoms can help protect against herpes, but of course, the best prevention is to avoid contact with an infected person. Prescription antiviral medications can be very effective if taken early, but they are expensive and don't work for everyone.

**Symptoms:** Groups of blisters followed by ulcerations. The blisters are usually preceded by stinging, itchiness, or general discomfort.

**Rx:** Take these supplements for up to 10 days.

| | |
|---|---|
| *Quercetin:* | Take 3000–4000 mg daily. |
| *Vitamin C:* | Take an additional 2000–3000 mg for a total of 5000 mg daily. |
| *Olive leaf extract:* | Take 2000–3000 mg daily (in a total of 4–6 capsules). |
| *Lemon balm ointment:* | Apply ointment gently to affected area up to 6 times daily. |

**WARNING:** Call your physician if the lesions do not heal after two weeks, or if they recur less than 2 weeks apart, or if they involve the eye. Herpes can cause blindness! Widespread blister eruptions may be a symptom of shingles and should be treated by a doctor.

### Ear Infections

Ear infections are one of the most common ailments of childhood. I think they are a rite of passage at summer camp! At one time, ear infections were routinely treated with antibiotics, but the overuse of these medicines has produced tenacious strains that are resistant to most common drugs. When a child gets an ear infection, parents often hear this advice: Be patient and wait it out. As any parent can tell you, that's not an easy thing to do when your child is in pain. I have found, however, that immunotics can shorten the duration of the infection as well as relieve symptoms. (Remember that bacteria don't care how old you are; ear infections can also strike adults.)

**Symptoms:** Pain in one or both ears often in conjunction with stuffy nose and fever. Parents should suspect an ear infection when an infant cries persistently, has a fever, and is generally irritable.

**Rx:** Take the following supplements for 5–7 days. If you are giving supplements to a child, only use powders mixed in fluid, liquid extracts, or chewable tablets.

| | |
|---|---|
| *Larch:* | Take ½–1 teaspoon in liquid 4 times daily. |
| *Echinacea:* | 1 dropperful every 2–3 hours or up to 2 (500 mg) capsules every 4–5 hours. |
| *Garlic:* | Adults can take 900 mg daily. Children can take 300 mg daily orally; or parents can apply commercial preparations of garlic oil directly into ear canal. (Do not use a cotton swab—use a dropper!) |
| *Olive leaf extract:* | Take 1000–2000 mg daily. |
| *Vitamin C:* | Take an additional 1000–2000 mg for a total of 3000 mg daily. |
| *Citrus bioflavonoids:* | Take an additional 1500 mg daily for a total of 3000 mg daily. |

**WARNING: Call your physician if you experience the drainage of thick mucus or blood from the ear, a loss of hearing, or a ringing in the ears. INFANTS UNDER SIX MONTHS OR WITH A FEVER SHOULD BE SEEN BY A PHYSICIAN.**

## Hepatitis (Viral)

Hepatitis is an inflammation of the liver most commonly caused by a viral infection. Since it can be chronic (especially type C), people with hepatitis must be vigilant about maintaining their liver health. There are five different hepatitis viruses (A, B, C, D, and E). Hepatitis A is spread primarily from the feces of a contaminated person. Poor hygiene is a major culprit, but it can also be spread through tainted food or water. Eating contaminated shellfish (exposed to raw sewage) is a common form of transmission. People catch hepatitis B through blood transfusions, the use of shared needles, and sexual activity. Hepatitis C, the most common form of hepatitis, has become a virtual epidemic. It is spread by sharing contaminated needles and by blood transfusions (blood is now screened for hepatitis C). In many cases, however, the route of transmission is unknown. Hepatitis B and D are often associated with the use of IV drugs and may occur simultaneously. Hepatitis E is spread like hepatitis A. So far, it is confined to third world countries and is not a problem in the United States. Some forms of hepatitis can either be acute or chronic. Hepatitis B, C, and D can all progress from the acute stage to a chronic disease that eventually destroys the liver. If you have ever had hepatitis or if you have chronic hepatitis, be kind to your liver! Obviously, excess exposure to alcohol, tobacco, and other toxins should be kept to a minimum. It is especially important to avoid acetaminophen, since daily use can cause liver damage.

**Symptoms:** Nausea or no appetite, vomiting, fever, malaise, joint and muscle aches, dark-colored urine, jaundice (yellow eyes and skin).

**Rx:** Take the following supplements for acute and chronic hepatitis. Acute hepatitis can last for several weeks, but chronic hepatitis can persist indefinitely. For acute hepatitis, take the highest dose. For chronic hepatitis, take the lowest dose. Hepatitis is a serious illness and shouldn't be treated without a physician. In addition to the Basic Immunotics Program, take the following:

| | |
|---|---|
| *NAC:* | Take 3000–6000 mg daily. |
| *MGN-3:* | Take 1000–3000 mg daily. |
| *IP-6:* | Take 6–9 capsules daily. |
| *Quercetin:* | Take 2000–3000 mg daily. |
| *Vitamin C:* | Take an additional 2000–3000 mg for a total of 5000 mg daily. |
| *Maitake D-Fraction:* | Take 2 dropperfuls daily. |
| *Curcumin:* | Take 1500 mg daily. |
| *Green tea extract:* | Take 1000 mg daily. |

**WARNING: If you suspect you have hepatitis, contact your physician. A blood test is necessary to confirm the diagnosis.**

## HIV (Human Immunodeficiency Virus) or AIDS (Acquired Immune Deficiency Syndrome)

HIV targets the immune system, making the body vulnerable to infections that are normally defeated with ease. Although there is no cure for AIDS, there are some new antiviral drugs that have proven to be remarkably effective in controlling the spread of the virus. Immunotics work in synergy with conventional treatments, providing much-needed immune support. HIV is spread through sexual contact, blood transfusions, and the sharing of contaminated needles. Keep in mind that it is much harder to treat HIV than to prevent it. Avoid HIV by practicing safe sex (not having sex with an infected individual and using a condom all other times) and never sharing needles. Today, blood is tested for HIV before it is used for transfusions; even so, if you are anticipating surgery, you can ask your doctor about donating blood ahead of time in case you need a transfusion.

**Symptoms:** Unexplained weight loss/loss of appetite; recurrent "opportunistic" infections such as shingles, oral thrush (yeast), molluscum, and pneumocystis pneumonia.

**Rx:** The Immunotics program for HIV is designed to enhance the effect of conventional antiviral drugs, not replace them. If you are HIV positive or have AIDS, it is imperative that you work with a knowledgeable physician. Take the following immunotics indefinitely in addition to the Basic Immunotics Program:

| | |
|---|---|
| *MGN-3:* | Take 2000–3000 mg daily. |
| *IP-6:* | Take 6–12 capsules daily. |
| *Colostrum:* | Take 9 (480 mg) capsules daily. |
| *Alkylglycerol:* | Take 1500 mg daily. |
| *Thymic protein:* | Take 3 packages sublingually daily. |
| *Garlic:* | Take 900 mg daily. |

| | |
|---|---|
| *NAC:* | Take 6000–8000 mg daily. |
| *Vitamin C:* | Take an additional 5000–9000 mg for a total of 10,000 mg daily. |
| *Curcumin:* | Take 1500 mg daily. |

**WARNING: If you suspect you have HIV, you must be evaluated and followed by a physician.**

### Influenza (Flu)

If it's winter, it must be flu season! Flu is a contagious respiratory infection caused by either a Type A or Type B strain of virus. The flu virus mutates from year to year, which is why it is important to get a flu shot each year. Although flu can cause great discomfort, in most healthy people it simply runs its course without complications. However, some 20,000 people die each year from flu; it exacts a steep toll among the elderly and immune-impaired population. Antiviral drugs may help speed recovery, but there is no effective cure. Immunotics can help your body kick out this uninvited guest faster and with less discomfort.

**Symptoms:** Fever, muscle aches, nausea, diarrhea, headache, stuffy or runny nose, and sore throat.

**Rx:** There is no cure for the flu, but the following supplements can help reduce symptoms and speed recovery. Full recovery usually takes 7 to 14 days. In addition to the Basic Immunotics Program, take the following:

| | |
|---|---|
| *NAC:* | Take 1500–3000 mg daily. |
| *Elderberry extract:* | Take 1 teaspoon every 3–4 hours. |

| | |
|---|---|
| *Western Larch:* | Take 1 teaspoon 3 times daily. |
| *Echinacea:* | Take 1 dropperful of tincture every 2–3 hours or up to 2 (500 mg) capsules every 4–5 hours. |
| *Garlic:* | Take 900 mg daily. |
| *Olive leaf extract:* | Take 2000–3000 mg. |
| *Vitamin C:* | Take an additional 1000–2000 mg daily. |
| *Citrus bioflavonoids:* | Take an additional 1500 mg for a total of 3000 mg daily. |

**WARNING: Call your physician if you experience a severe headache (especially with a stiff neck), shortness of breath (especially at rest), or rapid breathing, or if you cough up blood or thick, yellow, or green mucus or have a fever of over 102 degrees.**

### Pneumonia

Pneumonia is an acute infection or inflammation of one or both lungs. The next step beyond bronchitis, pneumonia results in the lungs becoming filled with liquid and is usually caused by a bacterial infection or a virus. Pneumonia should not be self diagnosed. A chest X-ray may be necessary to confirm the diagnosis, and antibiotic treatment is often required. But in many cases, immunotics can help give your immune system a fighting chance!

**Symptoms:** Fever, wet cough (with thick yellow or yellow-green mucus), and rapid breathing at rest.

**Rx:**  In addition to the Basic Immunotics Program, take the following supplements.

| | |
|---|---|
| *NAC:* | Take 3000 mg daily. |
| *Echinacea:* | Take 1 dropperful of tincture every 2–3 hours or 1–2 (500 mg) capsules every 4–5 hours. |
| *Astragalus:* | Take 1500 mg daily or 1 dropperful every 3–4 hours. |
| *Garlic:* | Take 900 mg daily. |
| *Citrus bioflavonoids:* | Take an additional 1500 mg (for a total of 3000 mg daily). |
| *Olive leaf extract:* | Take 2000–3000 mg daily. |

**WARNING: Persistent shortness of breath or difficulty breathing may necessitate hospitalization. CALL YOUR DOCTOR!**

## Postsurgery Recovery

During the weeks immediately following surgery, you must be especially vigilant about preventing infection. First, after surgery, the body must concentrate its efforts on healing the wound, depleting resources from the immune system. Second, despite elaborate measures taken to maintain cleanliness, the environment in which surgery is performed—a hospital or outpatient clinic—is often a breeding ground for infection. For these reasons, it is crucial for people to embark on surgery with a strong immune system and to make a special effort to support immune health following surgery.

**Rx:** To improve wound healing and prevent infection, begin taking these supplements 5 days prior to the operation and continue for at least 3 weeks after. These supplements will also help prevent the formation of blood clots, a major complication after surgery, but will not impair healing. In addition to the Basic Immunotics Program, take the following:

| | |
|---|---|
| *Colostrum:* | Take 9 capsules daily. |
| *L-glutamine:* | Take 1000–1500 mg daily. |
| *Alkylglycerol:* | Take 1500 mg daily. |
| *Probiotics:* | Take an additional capsule of Lactobacillus GG daily. |
| *OPC:* | Take 300 mg daily. |
| *Vitamin C:* | Take an additional 1000 mg daily for a total of 2000 mg. |
| *Curcumin:* | Take 1000–1500 mg daily. |

**WARNING: Prior to surgery, give your doctor a list of the supplements that you are taking. Postsurgery, call your doctor if you develop a fever or notice increasing redness surrounding the surgical wound, red streaks extending out from the wound, or increasing tenderness around the wound. Also call your doctor if the wound is draining pus.**

### Sinus Infection (Sinusitis)

Since I began practicing medicine 20 years ago, I have seen a dramatic increase in sinus infections. I believe this can be attributed to pollution. Constant exposure to toxins not only irritates nasal passages but also dampens the immune system's ability to fight off infection. Since viruses and bacteria thrive in the dark, moist nasal passages, once the infection takes hold, it can be very difficult to dislodge. To make matters worse, the overuse of antibiotics has led to resistant strains of bacteria that can cause sinusitis. Treatments that were once effective now don't work. Many people with chronic sinus infections have undergone sinus surgery, but all too often the infection comes back. My solution is to use the immunotics arsenal to clear out the congestion while giving the immune system a much-needed lift.

**Symptoms:** Sinus congestion and drainage with pressure and pain in the cheeks and around the eyes that worsens with forward bending, often accompanied by fever and  throbbing pain in the teeth.

**Rx:** In addition to the Basic Immunotics Program, take the following supplements for 1–3 weeks.

| | |
|---|---|
| *NAC:* | Take 3000–6000 mg daily. |
| *Echinacea:* | Take 1 dropperful of tincture every 2–3 hours or 1–2 (500 mg) capsules every 4–5 hours. |
| *Astragalus:* | Take 1500 mg daily or 1 dropperful every 3–4 hours. |
| *Garlic:* | Take 900 mg daily. |
| *Olive leaf extract:* | Take 4–6 capsules daily. |
| *Vitamin C:* | Take an additional 1000–2000 mg for a total of 3000 mg daily. |
| *Quercetin:* | Take 2000–3000 g daily. |

**WARNING:** Call your doctor if there is no improvement after 1–2 weeks of self-treatment, if you develop a fever of over 102 degrees, or if there is persistent bloody drainage or drainage of yellow mucus from the sinuses.

## Skin Infections

Although minor wounds—small cuts, punctures, and scrapes—usually heal on their own in healthy people, the risk of infection is always present. Therefore, it is important to properly care for a small wound before it becomes a bigger problem. The immunotics I recommend help the body heal from the inside out and the outside in; apply immunotics directly to the wound in addition to taking them orally. If you cut yourself on anything dirty, be sure to get a tetanus shot if you have not had one within the past five years.

**Rx:** In addition to the Basic Immunotics Program, follow this regimen for 5–7 days.

| | |
|---|---|
| *Tea tree oil:* *(10 percent strength)* | Apply directly to the wound 4 times daily. |
| *Echinacea:* | Take 1 dropperful of tincture every 2–3 hours or 1–2 (300 mg) capsules every 3–4 hours. |
| *Olive leaf extract:* | Take 3 (500 mg) capsules daily. |
| *Vitamin C:* | Take 2000–3000 mg daily. |
| *Garlic:* | Take 900 mg daily. |

**WARNING: Call your physician if you develop a fever, feel increasing tenderness around the wound, or notice increasing redness or red streaks extending from the wound or if the wound is draining pus. All of these are signs of acute infection and must be aggressively treated. Tea tree oil can cause allergic reactions in some people, which can be confused with infection. If in doubt, call your physician.**

## Sore Throat or Tonsillitus

A sore throat is caused by inflammation of the throat or tonsils, most often due to a viral or bacterial infection. Most minor sore throats associated with colds or flu do not warrant medical attention and are usually the result of a virus. If a sore throat is severe or is the primary symptom, you must visit your doctor for a throat culture to rule out strep throat, a condition requiring 10 days of antibiotics. If untreated, strep throat can lead to severe complications of the kidneys and heart.

**Symptoms:** Pain when swallowing; back of throat may be red and tonsils may be covered with "pus"; fever; swollen glands in neck.

**Rx:** In addition to the Basic Immunotics Program, take the following supplements for 10–14 days.

*Echinacea:*              Take 1 dropperful of tincture every 2–3 hours, dropped directly on tonsils or back of throat, or 1–2 (300 mg) capsules every 3–4 hours.

| | |
|---|---|
| *Astragalus:* | Take 1500 mg daily or 1 dropperful every 3–4 hours. |
| *Garlic:* | Take 1 300 mg tablet 3 times daily. |
| *Olive leaf extract:* | Take 2000–3000 mg daily. |
| *Vitamin C:* | Take an additional 1000–2000 mg (for a total of 3000 mg daily). |
| *Quercetin:* | Take 2000–3000 mg daily. |
| *Berberine:* | Take 3–6 capsules daily or 1 dropperful of tincture (usually found in combination with echinacea) 4 times daily, applied directly to back of throat. |

**WARNING: If you don't see an improvement within 3–5 days, call your doctor.**

## Stomach Flu (Gastroenteritis)

Although they usually run their course quickly, stomach bugs can be pure misery! They may strike alone or in combination with cold or flu symptoms. In most cases, antibiotics are worthless, but there are several immunotics that can help. Since you're losing so much fluid, it is important to prevent dehydration by drinking enough liquid. Of course, when you're feeling queasy, this is easier said than done. Try taking a few sips of apple juice or broth frequently throughout the day instead of trying to drink a full glass at a time.

**Symptoms:** Nausea and/or diarrhea, vomiting, fever and chills.

**Rx:** In addition to the Basic Immunotics Program, try these remedies for 3–5 days.

| | |
|---|---|
| *Colostrum:* | Take 3 (480 mg) capsules 3 times daily. |
| *Probiotics:* | Take an additional 2 capsules of Lactobacillus GG or an additional 2 teaspoons L. acidophilus. |
| *Berberine:* | Take 4 (500 mg) capsules daily or 1 dropperful of tincture 4 times daily. |
| *Garlic:* | Take 3 (300 mg) tablets daily. |
| *Aloe vera juice:* | Take 2 ounces 4–6 times daily. |
| *Grapefruit seed extract:* | Take 10 drops in 8 ounces of liquid 3 times daily (not to be used in the nausea and vomiting phase). |

**WARNING: Call your doctor if you have profuse, watery diarrhea or diarrhea lasting longer than 1 week, blood in the stools, or jaundice (yellow skin and eyes).**

## Stomach Ulcers

Ulcers are erosions that occur on the lining of the stomach or duodenum. At one time it was believed that ulcers were a result of excess stomach acid, but now we know that they are caused by the *Heliobacter pylori* bacterium. They can often be treated successfully with antibiotics, and I do not believe that immunotics are a substitute for the initial treatment. Immunotics, however, can be very helpful for preventing recurrences.

**Symptoms:** Burning or gnawing pain that worsens with an empty stomach. The pain is relieved by antacids, milk, or eating.

**Rx:** In addition to the Basic Immunotics Program, try these immunotics for 2–3 months.

| | |
|---|---|
| *Colostrum:* | Take 3 (480 mg) capsules 3 times daily. |
| *Probiotics:* | Take an additional 2 capsules of Lactobacillus GG (for a total of 3 capsules) or an additional 2 teaspoons of L. acidophilus (for a total of 3 teaspoons) daily. |
| *Berberine:* | Take 4 (500 mg) capsules or 1 dropperful of tincture 4 times daily. |
| *Aloe vera juice:* | Take 2 ounces of juice 4–6 times daily. |
| *Grapefruit seed extract:* | Take 10 drops in 8 ounces of liquid 3 times daily. |
| *L-glutamine:* | Take 1 teaspoon 3 times daily. |

**WARNING: Check with your physician if symptoms do not improve with antacids or if they persist for more than one month. You should not attempt to diagnose an ulcer on your own.**

## Yeast Vaginitis

Vaginal yeast infections are so common that about 75 percent of all women will get one at some point in their lives. Antibiotics are not only useless against yeast, they actually make them worse by killing off friendly bacteria in the gut that keeps yeast under control. Over-the-counter antifungal creams can be highly effective for yeast vaginitis, but if you have recurrent infections, immunotics can be especially useful.

**Symptoms:**  Itching, burning, whitish discharge.

**Rx:**  In addition to the Basic Immunotics Program, take these supplements for 5–7 days.

| | |
|---|---|
| *Garlic:* | Take 1200 mg daily. |
| *Olive leaf extract:* | Take 2000–3000 mg daily. |
| *Berberine:* | Take 2000 mg daily or 1 dropperful of tincture 4 times daily. |
| *Colostrum:* | Take 3 (480 mg) capsules twice daily. |
| *Probiotics:* | Take an additional capsule daily (for a total of 2 capsules) or an additional teaspoon of L. acidophilus daily (for a total of 2 teaspoons). |
| *Uva ursi:* | Take 1 dropperful of tincture 4 times daily. |

**WARNING: If yeast infections occur frequently (once a month or more) it is important to have a medical evaluation to rule out diabetes or another underlying cause.**

# EIGHT

# Foods to Strengthen
# Your Immune System

In chapter 3, I noted that micronutrient starvation is the leading risk factor for poor immune function. Ironically, in this land of abundance—where one out of five adults is clinically obese—too many of us are eating too little of the *right* foods. The end result? A deficit in important micronutrients that help to keep the immune system strong. The micronutrient gap not only makes you more vulnerable to common everyday ailments like colds and flus but over time increases your risk of developing such serious ailments as cancer, diabetes, and heart disease.

Fortunately, the micronutrient gap is easy to correct by making a few modifications in your diet. In this chapter, you will learn about powerful foods that can boost immune function—I call them *superfoods.* By adding them to your diet, you can make great strides toward improving your immune health. At the same time, I will alert you to *immune zappers,* foods that can dampen immune function. By reducing your intake of them, you can give your immune system a break. If you eat more of the good stuff and less of the bad, you can close the micronutrient gap quickly and easily.

## Food Can Be a Powerful Immunotic

Hippocrates, the father of modern medicine, said it best: "Food is the best medicine." He knew from personal observation that people who ate wisely tended to be healthier than those who did not. It took thousands of years, but we now know exactly why foods—or at least some foods—are such powerful medicine. Plant foods such as fruits, vegetables, and some spices like garlic and turmeric are a rich source of compounds called phytochemicals, natural disease-fighting substances that are key to helping the immune system do its job. There are thousands of phytochemicals, only a handful of which have been identified so far, and each has a unique benefit to the body. While we only have a partial understanding of phytochemicals to date, the more we find out, the more amazing these compounds seem to be.

Many immunotics sold as supplements are potent extracts of the same phytochemicals found in food. For example, you can get the same phytochemicals found in Asian mushroom supplements by eating fresh Asian mushrooms, albeit in lower quantities. The immunotic curcumin is derived from a group of chemicals extracted from the spice turmeric. You could eat curry powder to get the benefits of curcumin, but you'd have to eat an awful lot to get the same dose. Likewise, garlic pills are a concentrated form of fresh garlic. Eating a fresh garlic clove (mixed with a little bit of honey) is another way to obtain the healing power of allicin, one of the active phytochemicals in garlic.

You may ask, why can't I just take all my phytochemicals in a pill? Granted, you may get a higher concentration of a specific phytochemical in an immunotic supplement, but I believe that there is still great benefit to eating immunotic-rich foods, for several reasons. First, we know of so many different phytochemicals that it would be impossible to cover all the bases without taking hundreds of supplements daily. Second, I prefer dietary sources of micronutrients because foods contain complex mixtures of ingredients. Supplements, even natural ones, do not contain all of the components. The phytochemicals in food appear to work synergistically; if you isolate one or two you may not be getting the full benefit Nature intended. The best approach is to get as many nutrients as possible from the diet and make up any deficit with supplements, not the other way around. Where adequate intake is impossible, supplements are a must, and a godsend to optimizing body function. Still, a healthy diet lays the all-important foundation.

## The Superfoods

If you want to ensure that you are getting the full spectrum of immunotics found in nature, eat more fruits, vegetables, and whole-grain carbohydrates. Pay special attention to the superfoods, which are simply packed with immune-boosting power.

Think of the natural pigments found in fruits and vegetables as a key to their immune-boosting power. We find those brilliantly colorful yellow, red, orange, purple, and dark green fruits and vegetables attractive for a reason. A diet rich in them is associated with lower rates of cancer and heart disease. Just as a monochromatic painting is limited, so is a one-colored diet. To gain the full benefits of nature, make a rainbow of fresh fruits and vegetables your diet of choice.

Much of the benefit from these colorful foods comes from their skins or rind. However, concern about pesticides, waxes, and other preservatives means that buying organic produce is the way to go. Whatever you buy, wash your fruits and vegetables with a scrub brush or citrus-based produce wash to help reduce your exposure to pesticides and bacteria.

I know you've heard this before, but it bears repetition: Try to eat food that is as unprocessed and unadulterated as possible. Modern food-processing techniques strip food of important nutrients while adding a ton of unnecessary chemicals.

Although I am urging you to eat more plant foods, I am not suggesting that the only way to save your immune system is to become a vegetarian—not at all. There is no reason why you can't eat meat, chicken, and fish. If vegetarianism is the right choice for you, then go for it, but if not, keep in mind that much of our beef and poultry is contaminated with antibiotics and hormones, so I do recommend that you try to eat free-range, antiobiotic- and hormone-free meats and poultry. You can find these products easily in a well-stocked supermarket or natural foods store. As far as fish is concerned, pollution is also an issue. Try to eat fish caught in nonpolluted waters; in some cases, farm-raised fish is a better option. By the way, you can drive yourself crazy if you get too fanatical about this. If you travel a lot like I do, you may not always be able to eat organic or find free-range poultry or natural beef on a menu. Don't worry about it—just eat as well as you can when you are at home!

And now, on to the superfoods. Incidentally, it's hard to overdose on superfoods, so eat up.

### Allium Vegetables

**Superfoods:** Garlic, onions, chives, leeks

These mainstays of many tasty recipes have long been known to contain healing properties. Garlic in particular is rich in selenium, which provides the building blocks for an essential enzyme needed to make glutathione, an important antioxidant. It is also a heart-healthy food that prevents blood clots. The sulphur compounds in garlic have natural antibiotic and antifungal properties, and recent studies have shown that garlic can inhibit the growth of cancerous tumors. Garlic also appears to be useful in preventing prostate cancer.

Onions as well are rich in disease-fighting power. A study in the Netherlands showed that people who eat at least half an onion a day have half the risk of stomach cancer of those who don't eat onions at all. Why? Some believe that the ulcer-producing and cancer-promoting stomach bacteria *Helicobacter pylori* have a tough time surviving contact with the pungent sulfur compounds found in onions. Studies in Hawaii, China, Poland, and Italy have noted the same beneficial effects of onions, which also contain selenium.

### Berries

**Superfoods:** Blueberries, cranberries, blackberries, strawberries

Berries, in particular those that are rich in anthocyanidins, top the list of superfoods. Blueberries are my favorite. Not only do they taste wonderful, they are incredibly beneficial to the body. Loaded with phytochemicals like the anthocyanidins (which give them their blue pigment), blueberries help bolster the immune system. Blueberries contain natural antibiotic compounds, fiber, vitamin C, and flavonoids, all of which have been shown to be protective against cancer and other diseases.

These delicious little berries even help you battle mental and physical aging. Anthocyanidins appear to protect small blood vessels, such as those in the brain, from free radical damage. Their high content of pectin can also help lower blood cholesterol levels.

What about other berries? Well, black raspberries have reduced the incidence of cancer in rats fed a potent carcinogen. Although they are more difficult to find than blueberries, black raspberries are quite delicious and worth hunting for.

Cranberries offer many of the same benefits as blueberries. In fact, cranberry capsules are one of my recommended immunotics for urinary tract infections. Since most of us do not eat fresh cranberries, a glass of unsweetened cranberry juice daily is a good substitute. It's a good idea to read the label of whichever juice you choose. Many have more apple, pear, or grape juice than cranberry. Choose a juice that has the most cranberry you can find.

In addition to being great sources of vitamin C, strawberries and raspberries contain a natural antioxidant called ellagic acid (also found in cherries and walnuts), which is believed to have anticancer properties.

Make these tasty berries a mainstay of your diet. Use them

with whole-grain cereals for breakfast. Snack on them throughout the day. For dessert, try a nice bowl of fresh berries with a dollop of low-fat yogurt and a sprinkling of nuts. Or douse them with a dash of balsamic vinegar as the Italians do.

Citrus Fruits

**Superfoods:**  Oranges, lemons, tangerines, limes, grape-
fruits

The National Cancer Institute has cited citrus fruits as strong cancer fighters. As with many other foods, most of the benefits of citrus fruits are contained in the peel, so don't be too quick to discard it. Instead, wash it thoroughly and grate it liberally into baked goods, vegetable salad, fruit salad, or yogurt. Once again, buying organic makes it safer to use the peel. The white part of the grapefruit rind is particularly high in bioflavonoids, but it's bitter.

Carotenoid-Rich Foods

**Superfoods:**  Carrots, sweet potatoes, tomatos, pumpkins,
peaches, yellow squash, and dark green leafy
vegetables such as broccoli, romaine lettuce,
spinach

Carotenoids are a group of seven hundred different natu-rally occurring compounds in plants. Of this huge number, 60 are common in the food we eat—primarily strongly col-ored fruits and vegetables. As part of the Basic Immunotics Program, I recommend that everyone take an antioxidant complex with mixed carotenoids daily. But that's not enough—I also want you to eat a carotenoid-rich diet.

Carotenoids such as beta carotene, lutein, and lycopene

offer significant protection against lung, colorectal, breast, uterine, and prostate cancers.

The best known carotenoid, beta carotene, is a proven immune booster. In one study published in the *American Journal of Clinical Nutrition,* researchers analyzed the NK cell activity of 30 men, all of whom had been taking 50 mg of beta carotene every other day for 12 years. (The study was part of the larger Physicians' Health Study conducted by Harvard University.) The researcher found that the men taking the beta carotene supplements had significantly greater NK cell activity (about 42 percent) than those taking a placebo.

There are other less well known carotenoids that may even be better. Alpha carotene, for example, might battle cancer better than its beta cousin. To get this compound, eat your carrots. It's more concentrated in carrots than in any other fruit or vegetable, with the exception of pumpkin.

Lycopene, another unsung hero of the carotenoid family, is a potent antioxidant. Recent research tells a wonderful story: Lycopene helps fight prostate cancer and offers protection against bladder and pancreatic cancers. Some research suggests it can protect against heart disease. Lycopene is absorbed much better when it is cooked and combined with oil. Tomato paste and ketchup are better sources of lycopene than fresh tomatoes.

While dried fruits are also a good source of carotenoids, they are high in calories. Eat them in limited quantities as a snack food. (Some people are allergic to sulfites, an additive used to maintain color during the drying process. Look for sulfite-free dried fruits at your natural foods store.)

## Cruciferous Vegetables

**Superfoods:** Broccoli, cauliflower, Brussels sprouts, cabbage, kale, beet greens, watercress, collard greens, mustard greens, and Swiss chard

Yup. You need to eat your greens. Sorry. These vegetables contain many phytochemicals you can't get anywhere else, including sulforaphane and the indole-3-carbinols. These indoles are great cancer fighters. Studies at Rockefeller University have found that they protect against breast, cervical, and other cancers by inactivating harmful estrogens. These vegetables provide high concentrations of the carotenoids lutein and zeaxanthin (which may protect against macular degeneration) and are also good sources of beta carotene. Each of these vegetables offers a slightly different blend of phytochemicals; eat a wide variety of them for maximum immune power.

By the way, broccoli (and other vegetables) need to be chewed to release the beneficial indole-3-carbinols. Therefore, I don't recommend the powdered broccoli capsules that are being marketed to vegetable haters—they won't do the job. Instead, look for supplements that contain a processed form of broccoli that has already been converted into indole-3-carbinols. Of course, your best bet is to eat the fresh vegetable!

## Fiber

**Superfoods:** Soluble fiber—apples, apricots, bananas, oat bran, broccoli, psyllium

Insoluble fiber—grains, beans, celery, wheat bran, prunes

*Fiber* refers to food substances found in plants that contain no calories or nutrients and are not digested or absorbed by the body. While fiber sounds like a dietary big nothing, in fact it has enormous impact on your health. Numerous studies link a high-fiber diet to lower rates of cancer, heart disease, and diseases of the gut (such as spastic colon and diverticulosis.) Fiber comes in two varieties: soluble fiber (soluble in water) and insoluble fiber (not soluble in water). You need to eat ample amounts of both.

Insoluble fiber, abundant in whole grains, speeds up the movement of food through the body. In countries where fiber is a mainstay of the diet, there is far less incidence of colon cancer. Scientists believe that insoluble fiber helps to push toxic products out of the body that would otherwise build up in the colon.

Soluble fiber slows down the movement of food through the intestine, delaying the breakdown of starches to sugar, which causes a surge in insulin production. This can cause wild fluctuations of blood sugar levels that throw off your metabolism and can lead to insulin resistance and diabetes. Soluble fiber also binds to dietary fats in the intestines, preventing them from being absorbed and thereby lowering cholesterol in the blood.

Green Foods

**Superfoods:** Green drinks, spirulina

Fresh greens and green drinks (made from the juices of young, green plants such as barley and wheat grass) contain chlorophyll, a detoxifier of the body, a possible anticancer agent, and a good source of magnesium. Blue-green algae (such as chlorella and spirulina) also contain high levels of chlorophyll. These greens are abundant in antioxidants and other phytochemicals that protect plants from the same enemies that target humans, such as bacteria, viruses, fungi, and free radicals. The concentrated forms of green drinks are powerful immunotics. But don't think that this means you can skip your veggies—you still need to eat a wide variety of vegetables. Green drinks do not contain all the disease-fighting phytochemicals found in nature. They are, however, an easy and convenient way to bridge the micronutrient gap, especially on days when you don't eat right! Consider adding some spirulina or chlorella powder to your fruit drinks for an added boost to your nutritional arsenal.

### Asian Mushrooms

**Superfoods:** Shiitake, reishi, maitake, enoki

You've already heard a lot about mushrooms. In concentrated form, they can be powerful immunotics. You can also boost your immune power just by including some of these delicacies in your diet. As you know, Asian mushrooms in particular contain beta glucans, which "kick" the immune system into higher gear. Health benefits aside, these mushrooms are quite delicious grilled, sauteed with other vegetables, or wherever you'd use white mushrooms. If you haven't discovered the joy of Asian mushrooms, you are in for a real treat, and you won't have to travel that far. Asian mushrooms are now sold in the produce sections of major supermarket chains, specialty shops, and natural food stores. (I don't recommend traditional button mushrooms—some scientists think that they contain carcinogens.)

### Omega-3 Fatty Acids: The Good Fats

**Superfoods:** Cold water fatty fish like salmon, tuna, cod, and mackerel; deep green vegetables; flax; walnuts

For years, you've been told not to eat fat because it's bad for you, but now here I am telling you to go ahead and EAT FAT. As long, of course, as it's rich in omega-3 fatty acids. If you're like most Americans, you don't get enough omega-3 fatty acids in your diet. As you recall from the section on flaxseed, there are two kinds of essential fatty acids—omega-3 and omega-6. Most of us get enough omega-6 in our diet, but we are sorely lacking in omega-3. This deficiency places us at greater risk of cancer and heart disease. There is an easy solution—eat more fatty fish and other omega-3-rich foods. Try to eat at least three fatty fish meals a week (salmon, tuna, mackerel), if not more. Flaxseed and walnuts are also excellent sources of omega-3 fatty acids. Fresh flaxseed, which is growing in popularity, can be purchased in health food stores and ground in a coffee grinder. Sprinkle it on cereal, fruit, or yogurt daily. If you buy fresh flaxseed oil, keep it refrigerated in an opaque container, as it goes rancid easily. Here's yet another reason to eat your veggies—dark, leafy greens contain omega-3s, though not as much as fatty fish.

Soy Foods

**Superfoods:** Tofu, miso, tempeh, soy milk, soy protein isolate

Your immune system gets a big boost from soybeans and soy products. Soy is rich in antioxidants, phytochemicals, and isoflavones. The low rate of breast cancer in Asia, where soy products are a big part of the diet, led to studies in the West that showed that compounds in soy inhibit the growth of breast cancer cells. And there are other benefits for women as well. High levels of plant estrogens or phytoestrogens in soy cut down on the hot flashes associated with menopause. What's more, preliminary studies suggest that eating soy products may help retain bone mass and decrease the alarming rate of hip fractures (twice the rate of Japan) among older women in the United States. The phytoestrogens in soy can greatly reduce the need for hormone replacement therapy. Men aren't left out of the soy benefits: a major study of Japanese men in Hawaii found that higher consumption of tofu leads to a lower rate of prostate cancer. Even the FDA has gotten into the act; they now recommend soy protein as a food that lowers the risk of heart disease.

Soy is truly a miracle food. In addition to all of its benefits for the immune system and the body, growing soybeans has huge benefits for the earth. Fields of soybeans provide tons more protein than fields devoted to growing grasses to feed livestock. So you can take care of yourself and the earth at the same time.

I know, I know, you're probably thinking, "Yuck!" But tofu isn't what it used to be. Tofu—now available everywhere—is like a plain white canvas on which you can create the most amazing pictures. Taking on whatever flavors you add, tofu can be cooked with vegetables in a stir fry to taste like meat or marinated in wonderful oils, vinegars, and herbs and then simply grilled or even pan-fried (it tastes just like chicken). There are innumerable soy products on the market today that dress up simple soy and make it possible to include in many different parts of your diet.

Adding just a few meals a week of soy will go a long way toward boosting your health. It is also remarkably low in calories and very satisfying. For those who don't like soy foods, the powdered protein sold in health food stores is a good source of the beneficial phytochemicals found in soy.

Spices

**Superfoods:** Turmeric, cinnamon, ginger, rosemary,
              cayenne

Before the days of refrigeration, spices were more than just flavor enhancers; they were used to preserve food that would spoil otherwise. Of course, no one knew why spices worked so well, but today we know that many spices contain potent antioxidants and antimicrobial compounds. For example, according to researchers at Kansas State University, cinnamon can kill 99.5 percent of the bacteria in unpasteurized apple juice tainted with E. coli. Pass the mulled cider! Now imagine unleashing that powerful antioxidant and infection-fighting power in your body. Spices are some of the best-tasting immunotics around.

One of my favorite spices, ginger, is widely used in Asia to treat colds and stomach upsets. It is a terrific treatment for nausea, especially as a tea. The Japanese eat thin slices of ginger with sushi, a practice that may have been adapted to protect against microbial infection from raw fish. Grate ginger liberally into your stir-fries. Keep a box of ginger tea on hand to help reduce the misery of the common cold.

Turmeric has long been used in traditional Indian medicine. This tradition had it right! Turmeric, it seems, has anticancer activity, especially against colon cancer. Use turmeric whenever you want a dash of color in your meal (it makes a beautiful yellow) or to enliven soups, roasts, or any fish. Wash down with green tea! The phytochemicals in turmeric and green tea work especially well together.

Researchers at Penn State showed that the herb rosemary could significantly reduce the risk of breast cancer in rats.

Researchers fed the rats the same dried rosemary leaves sold at the supermarket. Sprinkle rosemary liberally into potatoes, marinades, and sauces.

Hot chili peppers also contain antioxidants (capsaicin is the most potent) and, despite their reputation for inducing heartburn, are actually good for digestion.

## Tea

**Superfoods:** Green tea is the best!

In many parts of the world, tea is an integral part of the daily diet and a ritual of life. Green tea contains compounds that the American Health Foundation found can protect against cancer. Studies in Japan have shown that people who drink a lot of green tea have significantly lower cancer rates than those who do not.

Antibacterial compounds in green tea called catechins are effective against *Streptococcus mutans,* the bacterial culprit responsible for tooth decay and gum disease. (This may be why Japanese parents for centuries have advised their children to drink green tea after eating a sweet.)

Green tea is more lightly processed than black tea, allowing it to retain more of its important phytochemicals. With about half the caffeine of a cup of coffee, it gives a nice morning wake-up to those trying to reduce their intake of caffeine. For the same reason, it's not your best tea choice before bedtime, but it can be delightful in the afternoon. Brew green tea lightly—for about half the time you would steep black tea. Any longer and it gets bitter.

# Watch Out for These Immune Zappers

Now that you know what foods are good for you, it's just as important that you know what foods you should avoid. The immune zappers listed here are foods that should be consumed in limited quantities. Unfortunately, many of them are the mainstay of the typical American diet! If you find a lot of these foods in your daily diet, the simple solution is to cut back gradually while adding more superfoods.

### Too Much Alcohol

Alcohol is a double-edged sword. Red wine is a good source of anthocyanidins, important immunotics. Moderate drinkers (1 or 2 drinks a day) tend to have lower levels of heart disease. However, there is some evidence that in women even moderate alcohol consumption can increase the risk of breast cancer. In excess, alcohol dampens immune function. If you drink, do so in moderation. If you have a history of alcohol dependency, a strong family history of breast cancer, or liver problems, steer clear of alcohol and consider taking the immunotic NAC to protect your liver.

### Cut the Carbohydrates

There are two types of carbohydrates: simple and complex. Simple carbohydrates include refined sugar, soda, white flour, and "junk" foods such as potato chips. Complex carbohydrates are found in fruits, vegetables, whole grains, and legumes. Simple carbohydrates break down very rapidly in the body, producing a quick surge of sugar into the bloodstream. Complex carbohydrates break down more gradually, providing a slow but steady stream of sugar.

A diet high in any form of carbohydrates—but especially simple carbohydrates—can raise blood sugar levels, leading to insulin overload. The hormone insulin helps glucose enter fat and muscle cells to provide the fuel that runs the body and makes our brains function clearly, but the body needs only so much glucose. The excess glucose has nowhere to go. It deposits itself as fat on the body, with the help of insulin, to be of use in a famine.

To add insult to injury, loading the body with sugar—either the sugar from the junk carbs or sugar itself from candy, soda, and too many desserts—also dampens immune function. Refined sugar decreases the activity of immune cells for several hours after it hits the bloodstream. This is why people who have diabetes are so prone to infection.

All these immune-zapping carbohydrates have their healthier counterparts. Refined white flour should be replaced by whole wheat. Brown rice is far superior to white rice, and sweet potato or yam is a much better choice than white potato. As for pasta, there are whole-grain varieties and pastas made from quinoa or Jerusalem artichoke (a member of the squash family.)

Having said this, I still want to caution against gorging on carbohydrates of any kind. ALL carbohydrates can raise blood sugar levels. The best way to prevent a surge in blood sugar is to always combine smaller amounts of carbohydrates with an adequate amount of protein. Put simply, your plate should contain more burger and less (or no) bun, more meatballs, less spaghetti, and more salmon (chances are, you're not eating enough fish anyway!) and less rice. And of course, pile your plate high with lots of colorful vegetables and fruit. An omelette is fine in the morning, but cut out the potatoes and eat whole-grain bread. By emphasizing protein more than carbohydrates, you're doing not only your immune system a favor but your waistline as well. Many overweight people find that eating higher amounts of protein and smaller portions of carbohydrates is the recipe for weight loss.

### Cured Meats

Hot dogs, salami, bologna, bacon, and the like are laden with chemicals and preservatives that are just plain bad for you. Nitrites that are used to cure meat form potentially cancer-causing chemicals called nitrosamines in your stomach. Fortunately, today there are chemical-free alternatives, such as natural beef, chicken, and turkey hot dogs, and nitrite-free bacon. Whenever possible, use these products instead of the nitrite-loaded ones. If you do eat a nitrite-treated food— if you can't resist that hot dog at the ballpark—wash it down with a glass of tomato juice. Antioxidant chemicals in tomatoes (including vitamin C) have been shown to block the formation of nitrosamines in the stomach.

### Transfatty Acids

I'll never know why they touted margarine as good for you! It is made from solidified vegetable oil, and in addition to hurting your immune system, it's murder on your heart! Margarine contains hydrogenated or partially hydrogenated fats. These fats are bad because they promote the formation of transfatty acids in the body, which raise blood cholesterol levels and increase the risk of breast cancer. If you use a breakfast spread, be sure to buy brands that specifically say they are free of transfatty acids. Butter in limited quantities is okay, but olive or grape-seed oil is better. Whole milk also promotes the formation of transfatty acids, so I advise drinking low-fat (1 percent) or non-fat milk. To avoid pesticides, hormones, and other toxins that can find their way into dairy products, buy organic milk. It's easy to find in health food stores and many supermarkets.

## Use the Power of Food

If you weigh the benefits of eating for immunity against the risks of disease and the side effects of antibiotics, it's easy to conclude that adding immune-boosting superfoods to your diet is your best bet. Treat your body the way Nature intended. Nourish it, fortify your immune system, and enjoy your long and healthy life. Every time you eat a fruit or vegetable—which I hope will be several times a day—you are gaining multiple benefits because the same foods that work to boost your immune system also help to prevent cancer and heart disease. Taking some time and making some effort to change your approach to eating will really pay off—not only in the long run in terms of your health and a more enjoyable old age, but right now as well.

Remember, the same food that is good for your immune system is good for the rest of your body as well. Eating for health makes your skin more luminescent and younger looking. Your eyes look clearer, and your vision is improved. It enhances your mental power while improving muscle tone and strengthening bones. Think of food as your medicine, and you'll go a long way toward preventing both disease and maintaining a strong, vigorous body.

# NINE

# Your Mind: A Powerful Immunotic

**P**hysicians and patients often ignore a powerful ally in the quest to maintain health and heal disease—the mind. My 20 years of practicing medicine have taught me that the human mind is a powerful immunotic, as powerful as any medicine. How a patient thinks—and, more important, *feels*—about illness, health, and the future can have a profound impact on his or her prognosis. The mind is as important a component of the Immunotics program as using immunotic supplements, eating well, and following a healthy lifestyle.

I'm not a victim of wishful thinking; there is hard science to back up my beliefs. In recent years, we have learned a great deal about the brain, the immune system, and how the two relate to each other. In the pages that follow, I will review some of the groundbreaking science in this area as well as show how you can use this information to your advantage. Learning to use your mind as an immunotic will not only help keep you well but is of particular benefit to those who are coping with chronic or serious illness.

Your mind can play amazing tricks on you—for better or for worse. It is so strong that at times our emotions can make a simple sugar pill work as well as any wonder drug! Laypeople are often surprised to learn that about 30 percent of the effectiveness of a particular medication or treatment is due to the so-called placebo effect, that is, if a patient *believes* a treatment will work, it does, at least for a while. For this reason, new drugs are tested in placebo-controlled trials in which neither the patient nor the physician know who is taking the real stuff—the so-called double blind study—because if either one knew who was getting the drug, it could influence the outcome of the study.

The placebo effect reinforces my assertion that our deeply rooted beliefs and assumptions are powerful medicine. Our beliefs are not simply fleeting emotions that run through our minds with little or no consequence. They trigger complex chemical reactions in the brain, which in turn impact virtually every cell in the body. Simply believing that a medication is effective could make our heart cells pump more efficiently or relieve joint pain, whether or not the medication actually works! In other words, the mind can effect physiology in very dramatic ways that we do not fully understand. There are many times when a patient with a cold or flu virus begs for an antibiotic (which of course won't do any good) when I wish I could simply prescribe a sugar pill. Of course, that wouldn't be ethical, but I do believe that for many patients it would speed up their recovery!

The flip side is also true; as I will discuss, there are times when our deeply held, subconscious beliefs can have a devastating impact on our health and well-being. My goal is to teach patients how to harness the power of the mind so that it works for them, not against them.

**Before I go on, let me make one thing very clear. I believe that the mind can enhance the effectiveness of both conventional and alternative therapies, but it is no substitute for medical treatment if you are sick. Relying on your mind as your sole treatment for serious illness can be deadly. You cannot cure cancer or AIDS with a positive attitude alone; you also need the appropriate medical therapy.**

I also want to clear up another misconception. When I say that the mind can have a profound influence on health, I am not suggesting, as some have, that negative thinking by itself can make you sick. Illness is not created out of thin air. On the other hand, I have no doubt that if the seeds of illness are already there—if you have the genes or the tendency to get sick—extremely negative emotions can make you more susceptible.

Likewise, I believe that one of the biggest hurdles in treating cancer or AIDS is the predominant belief in our society that these conditions are incurable. Although we may not have a cure per se for AIDS or for many cancers, there are many effective treatments for both of these ailments that can both extend and improve the quality of life. I make it a point never to label a patient as "incurable"—too often that becomes a self-fulfilling prophesy. If patients lose hope, they may not pursue all available options or take care of themselves in a constructive way. On the other hand, I have seen many patients who were given months or even weeks to live go on to defy the odds and remain alive years later. I have no doubt that if doctors were taught to think of these diseases as manageable conditions—and emphasized that belief to their patients—survival rates would be higher.

There is a poorly understood phenomenon in medicine called spontaneous remission, in which a seriously ill patient suddenly and mysteriously gets well. Medical science cannot explain spontaneous remission. Religious people would attribute it to a miracle or act of God. I have a hunch, however, that spontaneous remission will prove to be an example of the wondrous power of the mind—that is, many patients who beat the odds do so because they have learned how to create a healthy mental environment despite their physical problems.

The way patients view their lives and their illness can make the difference between life and death. A case in point is a patient I'll call Linda, whom I treated more than a decade ago for advanced breast cancer. After a mastectomy, Linda received a course of chemotherapy, but the cancer still spread. Linda came to see me after her oncologist had given her what Andrew Weil calls the medical hex—he told her that there was nothing more to be done. She didn't have, he said, more than a few months to live. After listening to Linda relate her grim prognosis, I smiled and asked her, "So tell me, Linda, what are your plans for the next five years?"

This is a question that I often ask my patients who are in the throes of a serious illness. I don't ask it to be cruel or unfeeling—I ask it because it forces people to refocus their thoughts on how they would be living their lives if they had not been diagnosed with their particular ailment. It helps them enlist their minds in the fight to get better.

Like many other patients in her shoes, Linda looked startled by my question. Everything in my tone and body language suggested that I believed that Linda was going to be around in five years even if her oncologist did not. I explained to Linda that no doctor—no matter how good—could accurately predict when a patient is going to die. The fact was, I had treated patients as sick as Linda who had gone on to live past the "expiration date" stamped on them by medical professionals. I also disputed the oncologist's assertion that there was nothing more that could be done, even though I did agree that there was nothing more that the oncologist could do. I promised Linda that I would help her manage her cancer through nutrition and powerful supplements that would help her immune system fight back. I told her that my program had worked well for many patients, but I was honest—I explained to Linda that I couldn't promise that she would live any longer. But . . . to get back to my question . . . just in case she did, what would she like to do with those extra years?

Linda smiled and for the first time looked alive. "Well, I want to spend more time getting to know my grandchildren, and I want to devote more time to my church community."

Linda had great plans, and I'm happy to say that she lived five more years to achieve them, and mostly in good health. Yes, eventually she did succumb to cancer, but not right away, and not before she had some wonderful years in between. It could have been a fluke that Linda beat the odds and survived significantly longer than expected, but I don't believe that. What I do believe is that Linda's survival is due to the fact that she embraced her life wholeheartedly. She gave her body the tools it needed to heal itself by eating well, getting enough rest, and taking some very effective immunotics. At the same time, Linda allowed herself to feel hope and optimism in her present and her future. I believe that Linda's life would have been considerably shorter, and certainly less fulfilling, had she not felt this way.

## Stress and Immune Function

It's easy to dismiss stories such as Linda's as mere coincidence or even pure hokum, but there's a rich body of scientific research to support the notion of the medical power of the mind. We know, for example, that when someone is under intense emotional stress, immune function measurably declines. Periods of extreme stress can result in lower NK cell, sluggish "killer T" cell, and diminished macrophage activity. In fact, widows and widowers are much more likely to get sick during the first year following the death of their spouse than their peers who have not experienced a major loss.

The first clue that stress could impact immune function was uncovered in the 1930s by Hans Selye, an endocrinologist who coined the term "stress" to describe feelings of anxiety and discomfort. As so often happens in science, Dr. Selye was investigating a completely unrelated topic—he was trying to learn about a particular hormonal substance that had been isolated from the ovaries of animals. In his now famous experiment, Dr. Selye injected one group of rats with the ovarian substance and the other group with a placebo. Several months later, he noticed some startling changes in the rats receiving the ovarian extract: They developed ulcers and severely impaired immune systems. At first, he believed that these changes must be due to the hormone shots, but much to his surprise, the rats receiving the placebo shots experienced the same changes! Dr. Selye had to rethink his hypothesis. If it wasn't the ovarian extract that caused the physical changes, what else could it have been? The only other factor affecting both sets of rats was the daily shots, which they all disliked. In fact, they hated the shots so much that often he had to hold down the rats to administer the shots while they writhed and squirmed to get away. Clearly, this unpleasant experience had exacted a steep physical toll.

Dr. Selye conducted other experiments in which he created equally unpleasant conditions for rats—holding them down for set periods throughout the day, plunging them in cold water, and the like. In each case, he duplicated the results of his earlier experiment.

Why would extreme emotional stress cause such profound and negative *physical* changes? Earlier I noted that thoughts trigger complex chemical reactions that affect many different body systems. It is similar in rats when they find themselves in an untenable situation. Their intense feelings trigger the stress response system.

When an animal or human being is under stress, the adrenal glands (located on the kidneys) produce stress hormones that ready the body for action. In humans, stress hormones raise blood sugar levels, speed up the heart rate, and send blood away from the gut to the legs—the "flight or fight" response. The stress response system dates back to primitive times when our human ancestors had to hunt down or fight off wild animals or combat unfriendly tribes as part of their daily existence. After a sudden burst of activity, levels of cortisol would drop, and their bodies would return to normal.

Our ancestors relied on the highly reactive stress response system to keep them alive.

Modern-day men and women experience stress differently from our ancestors. Since we no longer face the threat of being chased by wild animals, our stress is experienced in the workplace, on the highway, or even dealing with other family members. Our brains do not differentiate between these tamer forms of stress and life-threatening stress—any form of stress triggers the same response. Since we don't get to fight or flee, high levels of the stress hormone cortisol linger in the body. At high levels, cortisol is toxic and can damage various body systems—especially the immune system. Constant exposure to high levels of cortisol reduces the body's ability to fight off disease. That's why if you are under emotional stress, you should be sure to follow my immunotics stress regimen.

Stress has another, darker side. A highly stressful situation—the death of a spouse, the loss of a job, or a change in economic status—all too often triggers depression. Numerous studies have linked low mood or grief to the same kinds of changes in immune function seen in people under stress.

You can see that what helped us once can hurt us now; but today we don't have to be slaves to our primitive stress response system. We have excellent ways to deal with stress.

## It's a Two-Way Street

I imagine you're convinced by now that strong emotions can impact immune function, but you may be surprised to learn that the reverse also holds true. The health of and demands on your immune system can profoundly affect your emotional state. I see this every day in my practice. People who come to see me with very bad colds or flus often get sad and suddenly burst into tears for no apparent reason. Many of us understand this on an intuitive level; we dismiss our emotional behavior with "I'm not quite myself today." What we often don't realize is that our fragile emotional state is a result of a stressed-out immune system! Remember from chapter 2 that immune cells produce hormonelike substances called cytokines, which "talk" to other immune cells. This communication network keeps our responses coordinated and triggers particular immune responses. The immune system does not operate in a vacuum; it also communicates with nerve cells, digestive cells, muscle cells, and so on. It is closely linked to every body system, including the brain, the emotional center of the body. These systems are inextricably linked; it is difficult to tell when one ends and the other begins. In fact, a new field of science, psychoneuroimmunology (PNI), has emerged. This field explores the relationship among body systems. When we are sick, our cytokines send out alarm signals alerting the brain that we are under attack. The brain hears the distress call, triggering the stress response system. The combination of physical and emotional symptoms of illness can make us feel scared, emotionally vulnerable, and even depressed. It's easy to see how chronic illness can exact such a steep toll, physically and emotionally.

A particular form of stress is especially harmful because it can lead to a phenomenon called learned helplessness. Learned helplessness is induced by exposure to uncontrollable stressors—that is, finding oneself in a painful or very unpleasant situation from which there is no hope of escape. Numerous animal experiments have shown the effects of learned helplessness. For example, a rat is put in a cage in which it is exposed to a series of electric shocks or loud noises that it cannot escape. Later the rat is put in a diffrent cage where it can control the shocks. If the rat stays on one side of the cage, it will receive an electric shock, but if it moves to the other, "safe" side, it can avoid the shock. To make things even easier for the rat, a warning bell goes off alerting it that the shock is coming. This is a no-brainer even for rats! However, despite the fact that it can escape, this rat just sits there and takes the shock, making no attempt to move to safety. But if you put a fresh rat that has not had to endure previous shocks in the cage, it quickly learns how to avoid the shocks. Why can't rat number one learn the same lessons as rat number two? Based on its earlier experience, rat number one believes that it is powerless; therefore, it collapses and doesn't even try to find its way to safety. This is a prime example of learned helplessness in action.

Studies like these would be merely cruel if they did not reveal a deeper, more unsettling truth: Animals who develop learned helplessness are much more likely to get sick and die than normal. While many different types of stress—from loud noise to painful shocks to bright lights—can dampen immune function, situations in which the animal has no control—like the rat who can't escape from the shocks—produce far more dramatic declines in immune function and much higher rates of death.

For humans, feeling that you are out of control can be equally harmful. Several studies have linked a higher incidence of heart disease to people who have little control over their work, such as secretaries subjected to the whims of their bosses or air traffic controllers who are enduring the vagaries of air traffic patterns.

## Learned Optimism

Martin Seligman, the researcher who documented the effects of learned helplessness, has offered the antidote: learned optimism. Learned helplessness is the ultimate form of pessimism. People who feel helpless and out of control can only dread the future. But just as people can learn to be pessimistic, Dr. Seligman proposes that people can learn optimism and control. In his book *Learned Optimism: How to Change Your Mind and Your Life,* Dr. Seligman outlines a program that helps pessimists change their basic assumptions to a more upbeat, empowered view. Although Dr. Seligman's book is for a general audience, I feel it can be particularly helpful to people who are coping with illness or any other major life challenge.

Optimism is not merely a state of mind; it is also a reflection of action. People who are hopeful about the future—people who believe they have some control over their fate—will undoubtedly do more positive things for themselves. Maybe optimism is just a placebo, but then again, placebos can be powerful medicine! Your mind is an important component in maintaining your physical health. But I do believe that positive thinking only works when it is accompanied by positive action. Here are some tips I give my patients who are living with a chronic illness or under treatment for a serious illness.

***Don't focus on your illness.*** First and foremost, don't think of yourself solely as a patient or in terms of your illness. Your illness is but a piece of your life, not your entire life.

*Assume the best.* No one can predict the future, so you have as good a reason to believe that things are going to work out as to believe that they're not. Since optimists fare so much better, choose optimism!

*Don't put your life on hold.* Try to live as normal a life as possible. I don't suggest that you overtax yourself by running marathons or sky diving, but you should still incorporate things that you enjoy into your daily life. Yes, on days that you don't feel well, you should rest. But you can still plan vacations, see friends, go out to dinner, and do the things that make life rich and rewarding.

*Plan for your future.* Don't give up on your dreams—think about what you'd like to do over the next five (or ten) years, and begin to do these things. If you have always wanted to write a book, take a class in writing at a local college; if you always wanted to visit Maui, gather up travel books and plan your itinerary. Use your illness as a wake-up call to get moving!

*Get help.* If you are overwhelmed with negative thoughts, get some counseling. Counseling should provide emotional clarity and constructive problem solving, and of all the techniques I've encountered, I'm most impressed with neurolinguistic programming (NLP). Known as "software for the mind," NLP is a set of simple, straightforward processes that anyone can use to help their minds work better in conjunction with their emotions. Two books that I've found to be particularly helpful are *Beliefs: Pathways to Health and Well-being,* by Robert Dilts, Tim Hallbum, and Suzi Smith (Metamorphous Press), and *Heart of the Mind* by Connirae Andreas and Steve Andreas (People Press).

Some patients find that support groups consisting of people with the same problems are useful, but beware of the support groups that dissolve into a "pity party." The main reason for attending a support group is to share experiences and receive encouragement, not to wallow in despair.

Caring for your physical self and maintaining your emotional strength is essential to giving your body the immune-friendly home it needs. Your health and well-being depend on it.

# TEN

# Creating an Immune-Friendly Environment

Immunotics will, I hope, empower people to do all they can to maintain their health and vitality. Following the right Immunotics regimen for you, eating wisely, and taking care of yourself if you do get sick go a long way toward preventing serious illness.

But that's all wasted effort if you're trapped in a toxic environment. That undoes every good thing you do for yourself, so I'm going to ask you to review your lifestyle to make sure that you have done all you can to maximize the effectiveness of the Immunotics program in your everyday life, at home, at work, and at play.

## Is This Antibiotic Necessary?

You can protect yourself and your community against antibiotic resistance and chronically poor immunity by taking an antibiotic only when it is absolutely necessary. If your doctor is reluctant to prescribe an antibiotic for either you or your child, don't badger her until she gives in! Chances are, the antibiotic won't help anyway (it's either a virus, an antibiotic-resistant strain, or something your body does best to clear up by itself) and in the long run, could even hurt. You do have other options. Follow the Immunotics program for your particular problem. If you are really sick, here's some radical advice in today's world: Stay in bed for a few days. That's what sick days are for! Drink plenty of fluids and follow all those lessons your mother taught you when you were young. This will speed up your recovery better than any drug.

If you do need an antibiotic, take the full course of medication as prescribed. Do not discontinue taking the drug early without checking with your doctor. If you have to stop because of a side effect or allergic reaction, be sure to call your doctor immediately. When you discontinue taking an antibiotic in midstream, you are running the risk of creating an antibiotic-resistant strain. If the infection comes back, it will make it even more difficult to treat.

## Be Kind to Your Body

***Sleep is an immunotic.*** Simply getting enough sleep each night can make the difference between a great immune system and one that leaves you vulnerable to illness. Sleep is important for both emotional and physical health and is essential for immunity. If you miss even a single night's sleep, your immune system will suffer. In one recent study conducted at the San Diego Veterans Affairs Medical Center, it was found that a lack of adequate sleep for even one night can dramatically reduce NK cell activity the following day.

What constitutes a good night's sleep varies from person to person, but generally most people require from seven to nine hours nightly to feel fully refreshed.

Sleep serves two important purposes. In a broad sense, it gives our bodies time to recharge and refuel. Specifically, when our bodies are at rest, we place far fewer demands on our organ systems than when we are active and awake. This downtime gives our cells the opportunity to repair themselves and create new cells—including immune cells.

Not getting enough sleep is a major stressor. When you are exhausted, you feel overwrought and emotionally vulnerable. Your emotional state, combined with your sleep-deprived immune system, creates an environment within your body that is ripe for illness.

The only solution is more sleep! Unfortunately, that's easier said than done for many people. In the United States alone, some 50 million adults have some kind of sleep disorder. In fact, one-half of all adults over 65 suffer from sleep disorders. Some sleep problems stem from other physical problems—heart disease, alcohol abuse, adverse reactions to prescription drugs, depression, pain from arthritis, and even hormonal fluctuations associated with menopause.

Other sleep problems are rooted in poor habits. Human beings are cyclical animals; that is, our bodies work best when we are on a set schedule. In order to sleep well, go to bed at roughly the same time each night and get up at about the same time each morning. Too many people have erratic sleep habits. They sleep in on weekends (due to late nights) and struggle for wakefulness on workdays. Moreover, some people view sleep as a luxury, not a necessity, and deliberately stay up as late as possible. They wonder why they're so tired in the morning. Adjusting your schedule to make time for sleep can often "cure" many sleep disorders, but there are also some excellent natural remedies, such as valerian root, hops, and passionflower.

***Substance abuse.*** Excessive alcohol intake (more than one to two drinks daily) is harmful to your immune system! So are most illegal drugs, which, similar to alcohol, must be detoxified by the liver, depleting the body of glutathione. Our bodies have to deal with enough toxins in the environment without polluting them any further with unnecessary and dangerous drugs.

***The right amount of exercise.*** Moderate amounts of exercise can boost immunity, but too much exercise has just the opposite effect—it dampens immune function. By strenuous I mean continually overtaxing your body to the point of exhaustion—those of you who do it know what I'm talking about. Strenuous exercises depletes the body of antioxidants. People who overtrain their bodies are often magnets for every cold and flu that comes their way. There are times when you may be training for a specific event, such as a marathon, when strenuous exercise goes with the territory, but you shouldn't do it too often. When you are training hard, be sure to follow the Immunotics program for endurance athletes.

## Protect Your Children

No matter what precautions parents take, children will always get their share of colds, viruses, and common ailments. That's not necessarily a bad thing: The immune system "learns" how to fight disease from these early skirmishes with potential troublemakers. Of course, parents must protect their children from serious, life-threatening diseases while helping them develop the strongest immune system possible. It's a thin line to walk.

*Breast-feeding.* Breast-feeding is one of the best ways to give your infant's immune system a head start. The World Health Organization recommends breast-feeding your infant for the first two years of life. I understand that this may not be practical for working women who are out of the house a good deal of the day, or even for stay-at-home moms with other children and hectic schedules. I do believe, however, that you should try to breast-feed for at least the first six months. By then, your infant's naive immune system has had a chance to mature and will be better able to protect him or her from potential threats. In the meantime, you will be passing on important immune-boosting proteins to your infant that can only be obtained from breast milk. It's a once-in-a-lifetime opportunity for your child.

*Vaccinations.* It's become fashionable today for some advocates of alternative medicine—physicians and patients alike—to rail against vaccines for childhood diseases such as measles, smallpox, and whooping cough. They oppose vaccination on several grounds. First, they say that vaccinations can cause dangerous side effects. Second, they contend that vaccines are "unnatural" and that the body should fight its own battles. Without exposure to these serious pathogens, they claim, the child will grow up with a weakened immune system. Some people blame the epidemic of asthma on vaccinations! Finally, they say that vaccinations had little to do with the eradication of these diseases; rather, they say better hygiene is the reason why people are no longer dying of childhood diseases. As a result of this debate, many parents are reluctant (even scared) to give their children vaccinations. Parents should be much more frightened of the consequences of denying their children the appropriate vaccinations! Back at the turn of the century, it was common for a family to lose a child to disease. Today it is rare. Most Americans are spoiled—few of us have seen how childhood diseases can quickly cripple, maim, and even kill small children. But when I was working in Africa, I saw the deadly effects of tetanus, whooping cough, and other diseases that we rarely see today in the West. Sadly, in the remote villages where I worked, death for infants and children is still commonplace. All the soap and water in the world is no match for these deadly killers. Vaccines have saved millions of lives—quite possibly your own. Surely we don't want to turn back the clock to the days when our children's survival was left to fate.

As to the safety of vaccines, I've given them to thousands of children and have seen few problems. Granted, at one time, there were some reported adverse reactions to the old pertussis vaccine, but that vaccine is rarely used. The new vaccine has not caused the same side effects. Similarly, the live oral polio vaccine is being replaced by a much better form that is inactivated, thus unable to cause polio.

Children should receive vaccinations against chicken pox, diphtheria, mumps, whooping cough, measles, polio, tetanus, hepatitis B, *Hemphilus influenza* type B, and German measles. If your child has asthma or a chronic illness, your doctor may also recommend an annual flu shot.

***Don't go overboard.*** Although no one would recommend exposing young infants to contagious diseases, it is equally ridiculous to raise children in a "squeaky clean" environment. The immune system learns through experience; it needs to be exposed to a wide range of microorganisms. Trying to keep a child in a sterile environment can be harmful. Recently, many toy manufacturers have added Microban, a product similar to the active ingredient in antimicrobial soaps, to children's toys, toothbrush handles, high chairs, and crib blankets. It's even being used in cutting boards and on steering wheels in Japan. I seriously doubt the necessity or wisdom of using these products. First of all, they are ineffective against viruses, the cause of colds and flus. Second, these products could give rise to resistant strains of microbes. Finally, the overuse of antimicrobial products undermines your child's immune system by denying it an opportunity to learn how to deal with bacteria and other microbes normally found in the environment. Overprotecting your child from mild bugs may leave her unable to defend herself when serious ones come around. If you really want your child to stay healthy, teach him to wash his hands well with ordinary soap and water after playing with other children and before meals.

*Be realistic.* Parents need to understand that even under the best of circumstances, children will catch their share of colds, viruses, and ear infections. It is unrealistic to expect a child never to get sick or miss a day of school. Many parents mistakenly believe that giving a child an antibiotic is the way to cure everything. I can understand; who wants to see their child suffer while they can do what seems like nothing at all? You *can* do something. When a child gets sick, there is no substitute for bed rest and proper care. Sending a sick child to school harms the child and endangers the other kids in the class. If you work, be sure to have a contingency plan if your child needs to stay home.

## Kitchen Safety Tips

Taking a few simple precautions in the kitchen can have a dramatic impact on your health and the health of your family.

*Beware of the kitchen sink.* The wet, moist environment of the kitchen sink provides a perfect breeding ground for bacteria. Wet rags and sponges are the worst culprits! Dry them thoroughly between each using, and dispose of them frequently. Be extra careful when someone is sick. If you wipe off the sick person's plate with a sponge, you are giving those bacteria a wonderful place to grow. If you use the same sponge to wipe up other dishes or the kitchen table, you spread the bacteria around. Avoid these problems by wiping the plate with a disposable paper towel or throwing the sponge away after it comes in contact with the plate. I go to a discount store and buy dozens of sponges at a time because I use them up so quickly!

*Cutting boards.* To avoid cross-contamination of meat and produce, use a separate cutting board for each. Be sure to clean thoroughly with warm soap and water any surface that may have come in contact with raw meat, poultry, or chicken, including your hands. (Wood cutting boards are better than plastic because they are easier to clean. Plastic boards have little nooks and crannies that can harbor bacteria.) I recommend that you wash down the cutting board you use for meat at least once a week with a dilute solution of bleach and water.

*Cook your meat thoroughly.* Undercooked beef or poultry can spread salmonella and E. coli infection. Cook beef and poultry until the juices run clear, or check it with a meat thermometer. Do not eat chicken unless it is cooked thoroughly—if chicken is still pink inside, it is underdone. Undercooked ground meat is a particular problem—do not eat rare (red on the inside) hamburgers, especially in restaurants.

*Rinse produce carefully.* Try to buy organically grown, pesticide-free produce. You may want to consider a special produce cleaner. I use one called Fit Spray made by Proctor and Gamble; there are many others.

## Reduce Your Exposure to Toxins

There is no way to avoid all toxins. They are everywhere—in the air, in our food, even in our water. Fortunately, the human body has an elaborate system to detoxify potentially hazardous substances before they can do damage. However, I believe we are overtaxing that system. Remember that many of the chemicals we are exposed to on a daily basis—from secondary cigarette smoke to smog to pesticides—promote the formation of free radicals in the body, which not only promotes disease but hurts immune cells, too.

If possible, reduce your exposure to toxins. Since chlorine or other contaminants, such as lead, can find their way into tap water, I recommend drinking filtered water. There are many excellent water purification systems on the market, from pitchers to whole-house systems. Considering the cost of bottled water, even the most expensive of these are a good investment.

Try to use products that are free of unnecessary dyes and other chemicals as much as possible. You can purchase natural unbleached paper goods and nontoxic kitchen cleaning supplies at health food stores and even in some supermarkets. These products are not only better for you, they are better for the environment.

Avoid exposure to any unnecessary toxins at work. Do you work near a piece of equipment such as a copy machine that could be giving off irritating fumes? If so, ask to have it moved away from your work area.

The use of insecticides is another big issue, especially for homeowners. To avoid potential toxins in insecticides, many homeowners are switching to organic gardening methods.

Even if you are careful with insecticides, your neighbors may not be. Therefore, ask them ahead of time to notify you before they use insecticides. Those of you at a high risk of cancer may decide to stay inside or even spend a night or two away from home to avoid the exposure.

## Protect Yourself in High-Risk Situations

You could be at high risk if you work in a poorly ventilated office building, are the parent of a small child, work in a hospital, are a school teacher, or travel on mass transit, especially during cold and flu season. In addition to following the Immunotics program for high-risk situations, here are some simple ways to reduce your risk.

*Get a flu shot.* The rule of thumb is that anyone over the age of 60, pregnant women, and people with cardiac or respiratory problems must have a flu shot. I also recommend it to people who are at high risk of getting the flu, such as health care workers, school teachers, and those who travel on airplanes or mass transit. I take one each year myself. Even if you don't fall into any of these high-risk groups, you may want to get a flu shot. It is the best way to protect yourself against the flu.

Influenza is caused by a virus of the genus *orthomyxovirus.* Although we may treat it casually, it is not a trivial problem—flu accounts for up to 20,000 deaths each year in the United States. And that's in a normal year. Some flu strains are worse than others. The great flu pandemic of 1917–1919—the so-called Spanish or swine flu—killed up to 40 million people worldwide. During World War I more soldiers died of the flu than of battle wounds.

*Fresh air.* Fresh air is a great antidote to infection! Wherever possible, open windows, even in the winter. Don't allow rooms to get overheated and stuffy—that's perfect breeding ground for colds and flus. Of course, it is not always possible to open the windows, especially in closed office buildings where the windows are sealed to save on energy costs. If you work in a closed office building, you must assume that you are being exposed to every cough, cold, and flu in the office! I work in a closed building, and obviously I am exposed to sick people. To fight back, I run an ionizer and air purifier all day to clean the air next to my desk. An ionizer/purifier draws pollutants, allergens, and viruses out of the air and away from you. There are many brands on the market, but be sure to buy one with a HEPA filter. Of course, nothing will protect you completely from airborne bacteria and viruses, but an ionizer/purifier can at least reduce your exposure. In addition, badger your building maintenance department to make sure that the duct work is clean and the air filters are functioning properly.

*Be aware of your surroundings.* If you work in an environment where people are frequently sick, avoid coming in contact with places of likely contamination. Don't use someone else's telephone if you know he or she is sick. Beware of doorknobs, especially in the bathroom. If someone coughs or sneezes, the airborne microbe will often land on the doorknob and end up on your hand, where it can spread if it comes in contact with your nose, mouth, or eyes. During cold or flu season, don't touch the doorknobs directly; push open a door with your arm or, if you can't avoid the doorknob, protect yourself by opening it with a paper towel. I know this sounds silly, but it can dramatically reduce your chances of getting sick.

*Hospital workers.* Hospital workers must be especially vigilant about washing their hands often. Hospitals are the only place where using antibiotic soap is an absolute necessity. Be mindful that any surface you come in contact with is potentially infected. Minimize contact with contaminated surfaces (doorknobs, elevator buttons, etc.), and always wash your hands thoroughly before you eat.

*Teach children to wash their hands.* Whether at home or at school, there is no better way to prevent infection than frequent hand washing. To make it easy for kids, teachers should provide Handiwipes for children in the classroom so they can wash up before snacks and lunch. Parents should make hand washing a regular routine at home.

## Travel Tips

*Airplanes.* Being in an airplane poses an even greater risk than working in a closed building; not only are you at the mercy of a central ventilation system, but the air is recycled, redistributing airborne germs throughout the cabin. If you are sitting near a person who is sick, the odds are even greater that you will catch it. So what do you do? If you find that you always get sick after an airplane flight, put yourself in high-risk mode before your trip. Follow the Immunotics program for people in a high-risk environment; be sure to get enough sleep and give yourself a day or two to recover after the flight. If you have a serious immune deficiency problem, such as AIDS, or are taking an immunosuppressant drug, consider wearing a mask on the plane. If you are flying during flu season, get a flu shot. If you are flying into another time zone, be sure to get enough rest! Remember the importance of sleep, and drink plenty of nonalcoholic fluids on the plane.

***Overseas travel.*** First and foremost, if you are traveling to a foreign country, make sure that your vaccinations are up to date. This is the best way to prevent contracting a serious, life-threatening disease.

If you are visiting a third world country or a place where the water or sanitation is problematic, be vigilant about protecting yourself! Follow my Immunotics program for travelers. But you also need to take special precautions so that you don't get sick.

Don't drink the tap water . . . ever. Stick to bottled water, even when you are brushing your teeth. Be especially careful about swallowing water when you shower. Of course, local people may tell you that the water is fine because they never get sick from it. That may be true, but their bodies have had a lifetime to develop an immunity to the microbes in the water. The same organisms that are harmless to them can cause great harm to you.

Never, never eat anything from a street vendor—it is a sure way to get sick. Try to eat in hotels and restaurants that cater to tourists, but don't let your guard down. Many foreign countries do not have the same system of monitoring the cleanliness of restaurants as we do in the United States. Don't take anything for granted. Don't eat any raw fruits, vegetables, or fresh salads. Make sure that your food is thoroughly cooked. Beware of hidden sources of tainted water. For example, if a waiter brings a wet plate to the table, be sure to dry it off thoroughly before putting food on it, and be sure to ask for your drinks without ice.

## Outdoor Tips

I love to spend time outdoors hiking and camping. But there are two things outdoor enthusiasts need to watch out for— sunburn and bug bites.

*Avoid too much sun.* Moderate amounts of sun (in small doses) is good for you, but excessive exposure to sun can depress your immune system. Sunscreens are helpful in preventing sunburns, but they deceive us into spending more time in the sun than we should. Even with sun protection, avoid exposure during the peak hours (10 A.M.–2 P.M.). When you are out during peak hours, wear a hat to protect your face.

*Use bug repellent.* As of this writing, there have been some reported cases of mosquito-borne viruses in New York. And in many parts of the country, Lyme disease, which is spread by deer ticks, is a major concern. I recommend using a natural bug repellent made from soybean oil called Bite Blocker. Use it on any open skin and on clothing. Bite Blocker is made by a company called

Consep, in Bend, Oregon. There are others on the market; this one has worked for me and does not have the unpleasant odor found in citronella-based products.

The key to getting well and staying well is simple. Give your immune system the tools it needs to do its job, and it will do it—and it will do it better than any drug, treatment, or therapy that medicine can dream up. Work with your immune system and it will work *for* you, not against you.

If you get sick a lot, don't assume your immune system is at fault. Take stock of your lifestyle. Ask yourself, what are you doing that is hampering your immune system from doing the work that Nature intended? You can't run yourself into the ground, eat a poor diet, neglect your health in other ways, and then expect your immune system to pick up the slack. Sorry. It doesn't work that way. You are an important part of this process, and the more you do, the better the result.

It doesn't take that much to keep your immune system in tip-top condition. Taking your immunotic supplements daily is a simple but powerful way to recharge your immune system. Adding superfoods to your diet is an easy (and delicious) way to feed your immune system the fuel it needs to keep running. And don't forget the importance of sleep, fresh air, and moderate exercise. These small things can reap huge results in terms of improved health and well-being.

If you do get sick (as we all do), use immunotics to speed up your recovery. But remember that immunotics can't do the job alone; they work best when you work with them.

Within the pages of this book is the blueprint for a healthy, vital life. Use it in good health!

# Resources

The following list includes some of the high-quality natural products that I prescribe to my patients. If you are unable to find them at your local health food store, you can call the distributor or manufacturer directly.

*Acidophilus powder*
Ethical Nutrients/
Metagenics
1-800-692-9400
Supplier Of Ultradophilus

*Alkylglycerol*
Scandanavian Naturals
1-800-288-2844

*Aloe Vera*
Light Resources Unlimited
1-800-760-3530
Distributor of Carrington
Laboratories aloe vera mucopolysaccharide extract

*Astragalus*
Nature's Way
1-800-9-NATURE

*Berberine*
Enzymatic Therapy/
Phyto-Pharmica
1-800-553-2370

*Beta Glucan*
Immunocorp.
Supplier of Norwegian
Beta Glucan
1-800-446-3063, ext. 100

*Colostrum*
Symbiotics Corporation
1-800-784-4355
Supplier of New Life
Colostrum powder and
capsules

*Cranberry*
Cran-Actin by Solaray
1-800-669-8877

*Curcumin*
Jarrow
1-800-726-0886

*Echinacea*
Eclectic Institute
1-800-332-4372

*Flaxseed*
Omega Nutrition
1-800-661-3529
Supplier of Hi-Lignan
Nutri-Flax

*Garlic*
Ethical Nutrients/
Metagenics
1-800-692-9400

*Grapefruit Seed Extract*
NutriBiotic
1-800-785-9791

*Green Tea Extract*
Jarrow
1-800-726-0886

**IP-6**
Enzymatic Therapy/
Phyto-Pharmica
1-800-553-2370
Supplier of Cellular Forte

**Lactobacillus GG**
CAG Functional Foods
1-888-828-4242
Supplier of Culturelle

**Larch**
Eclectic Institute
1-800-332-4372
Supplier of Larix brand
Western Larch powder

**Lemon Balm**
Enzymatic Therapies
1-800-553-2370
Supplier of Herpilyn

**L-Glutamine Powder**
Advanced Medical Nutrition
1-800-654-4432

**Olive Leaf**
Eastpark Research
1-702-837-1111

**Maitake D-Fraction**
Maitake Products
1-800-332-4372

**MGN-3**
Lane Labs
1-800-526-3005

**Mushroom Extracts**
Planetary Formulas
1-800-777-5677

**7 KETO DHEA**
Enzymatic Therapies
1-800-553-2370

**Tea Tree Oil**
Eclectic Institute
1-800-332-4372

**Thymic Protein A**
Klabin Marketing (from
Longevity Research)
1-800-933-9440

**Uva Ursi**
Vitamin Research, Inc.
1-800-877-2447

# Bibliography

"Antimicrobial Resistance: Data to Assess Public Health Threat From Resistant Bacteria are Limited." United States General Accounting Office Report to Congressional Requesters, April 1999.

Babal, K. "Thymic Protein May Enhance Immunity." *Nutrition Science News* 3 (1998): 578–80.

Barilla, Jean, ed. *The Antioxidants.* New Canaan, CT: Keats, 1995.

Beardsley, T. R., M. Pierschbacher, and G. D. Wetzel. "Induction of T-cell Maturation by a Cloned Line of Thymic Epithelium." *Proceedings of the National Academy of Sciences* 80 (1983): 6005–09.

Bendich, A., and L. Langseth. "The Health Effects of Vitamin C Supplementation: A Review." *Journal of the American College of Nutrition* 14: 124–36.

Ber, L. "Yeast-Derived Beta-1,3-D-Glucan: An Adjuvant Concept." *American Journal of Natural Medicine* 4 (1997): 21–25.

Blumenthal, Mark. "Echinacea Study Misreported in Press." *Whole Foods,* January 1999, pp. 45–50.

Brack, C. E. "N-acetylcysteine Slows Down Aging and Increases the Life Span of *Drosophila melanogaster.*" *Cellular and Molecular Life Sciences* 53: 960–66.

Brodsky, James. "Echinacea: Continuing Education Module." *Nutrition Science News,* February 1999, pp. 1–8.

Brohult, A., J. Brohult, S. Brohult, et al. "Effect of Alkoxyglycerols on the Frequency of Fistulas Following Radiation Therapy for Carcinoma of the Uterine Cervix." *Acta Obstetricia Gynecologica Scandinavica* 58 (1979) 203–7.

Brohult, A., J. Brohult, S. Brohult, et al. "Reduced Mortality in Cancer Patients After Administration of Alkoxyglycerols." *Acta Obstetricia Gynecologica Scandinavica* 65(1986): 779–85.

Castell, L., and E. Newsholme. "Glutamine and the Effects of Exhaustive Exercise Upon the Immune Response." *Canadian Journal of Physiology and Pharmacology* 76 (1998): 524–32.

Challem, Jack. "NAC: Your Best Cold and Flu Defense." *Let's Live* 42 (1998): 45.

Chandra, R. K. "Graying of the Immune System: Can Nutrient Supplements Improve Immunity in the Elderly?" *JAMA* 277 (1997): 1398–99.

Chang, A., M. Lotze, and D. Pardoll. "Mobilizing the Body's Defenses Against Cancer." *Patient Care,* March 30, 1996, pp. 32–49.

Cichoke, A. "Maitake: The King of Mushrooms." *Townsend Letter for Doctors* 130 (1994): 432–33.

Clinton, S. K. "Lycopene: Chemistry, Biology, and Implications for Human Health and Disease." *Nutrition Reviews* 56 (1998): 35–51.

De Flora, S., C. Grassi, and L. Carati. "Attenuation of Influenza-like Symptomatology and Improvement of Cell-Mediated Immunity with Long-term N-acetylcysteine Treatment." *European Respiratory Journal* 10 (1997): 1535–41.

DuPont, H. L. "Lactobacillus GG in Prevention of Traveler's Diarrhea: An Encouraging Step." *Journal of Travel Medicine* 4 (1997): 1–2.

"Flax Facts." *Journal of the National Cancer Institute* 83 (1991): 1050–52.

Fulder, S., and J. Blackwood. *Garlic: Nature's Original Remedy.* Rochester, VT: Healing Arts Press, 1991.

Ghoneum, M. "Anti-HIV Activity in Vitro of MGN-3, an Activated Arabinoxylane from Rice Bran." *Biochemical and Biophysical Research Communications* 243 (1998): 25–29.

———. "Enhancement of Human Natural Killer Cell Activity by Modified Arabinoxylane from Rice Bran (MGN3)." *International Journal of Immunotherapy* 14 (1998): 89–99.

Goleman, D., and J. Gurin. *Mind Body Medicine.* Yonkers, NY: Consumer Reports Books, 1995.

Gorbach, S. L. "Efficacy of Lactobacillus in Treatment of Acute Diarrhea." *Nutrition Today Supplement* 31 (1996): 2S–4S.

Graf, E., and J. W. Eaton. "Antioxidant Functions of Phytic Acid." *Free Radical Biology and Medicine* 8 (1990): 61–69.

Hamilton, G. "Let Them Eat Dirt." *New Scientist,* July 18, 1998.

Hauer, J., and F. A. Anderer. "Mechanism of Stimulation

of Human Natural Killer Cytotoxicity by Arabinogalactan from *Larix occidentalis.*" *Cancer Immunology and Immunotherapy* 36 (1993): 237–44.

Jaret, P. "The Antibiotic Crisis." *Hippocrates* 12 (1998): 26–33.

Jones, C. "Aloe: More Than Skin Care." *Nutrition Science News* 3: 398.

Julius, M., C. A. Lang, L. Gleiberman, et al. "Glutathione and Morbidity in a Community Based Sample of Elderly." *Journal of Clinical Epidemiology* 47 (1994): 1021–26.

Kelly, G. "Clinical Applications of N-acetylcysteine." *Alternative Medicine Review* (1998): 114–27.

Kubo, K., and H. Nanba. "The Effect of Maitake Mushrooms on Liver and Serum Lipids." *Alternative Therapies in Health and Medicine* 2 (1996): 62–66.

Lapcevic, J. "A New Biologically Active Thymic Protein to Stimulate Cell-Mediated Immunity." *Townsend Letter for Doctors and Patients,* February/March 1997.

Lau, B. *Garlic for Health.* Wilmot, WI: Lotus Light Publications, 1988.

McCaleb, Rob. "Aloe Vera Compound Effective Against Mouth Ulcers." *Herbalgram* 32:12.

Melchart, D., K. Linde, F. Worku, et al. "Immunomodulation with Echinacea: A Systematic Review of Controlled Clinical Trials." *Phytomedicine* 1 (1994): 245–54.

Messina, M., and S. Barnes. "The Role of Soy Products in Reducing Risk of Cancer." *Journal of the American Dietetic Association* 91 (1991): 836–40.

Meydani, S. N., M. Meydani, J. Blumberg, et al. "Vitamin E Supplementation and in Vivo Immune Response in Healthy Elderly Subjects." *JAMA* 277 (1997): 1380–86.

Michnowicz, Jon, and H. L. Bradlow. "Inductions of Estra-

diol Metabolism by Dietary Indole-3 Carbinol in Humans."
*Journal of the National Cancer Institute* 82 (1990): 947b–49b.

Morales, A. J., J. J. Nolan, J. C. Nelson, et al. "Effect of Replacement Dose of DHEA in Men and Women of Advancing Age." *Journal of Clinical Endocrinology Metabolism* 78 (1994): 1360–67.

Mowrey, D. *Next Generation Herbal Medicine.* New Canaan, CT: Keats, 1990.

Nagabhushan, M. "Curcumin as an Inhibitor of Cancer." *Journal of the American College of Nutrition* 11 (1992): 192.

Nanba, Hiroaki. "Antitumor Activity of Orally Administered 'D-fraction' from Maitake Mushroom (*Grifola frondosa*)." *Journal of Naturopathic Medicine* 4: 10–15.

Nyquist, A. C., R. Gonzales, J. Steinder, et al. "Antibiotic Prescribing for Children with Colds, Upper Respiratory Tract Infections, and Bronchitis." *JAMA* 279 (1998): 875–77.

Ohno, N., K. Iino, T. Takeyama, et al. "Structural Characterization and Antitumor Activity of the Extracts from Matted Mycelium of Cultured *Grifola frondosa.*" *Chemical and Pharmaceutical Bulletin* 33 (1985): 3395–3401.

Oksanen, P., S. Salminen, M. Saxelin, et al. "Prevention of Traveler's Diarrhea by Lactobacillus GG." *Annals of Medicine* 22 (1990): 53–56.

Packer, L., and C. Colman. *The Antioxidant Miracle: Your Complete Plan for Total Health and Healing.* New York: Wiley, 1999.

Packer, L., and J. Fuchs. *Vitamin C in Health and Disease.* New York: Marcel Dekker, 1997.

Passwater, R. A., and C. Kandaswami. *Pycnogenol: The Super "Protector" Nutrient.* New Canaan, CT: Keats, 1994.

Penn, N. D. "The Effect of Dietary Supplementation with

Vitamins A, C and E on Cell Mediated Immune Function in Elderly Long Stay Patients: A Randomized, Controlled Study." *Age and Aging* 20 (1991): 169–74.

Plemons, J. M., T. D. Reps, W. H. Binnie, et al. "Evaluation of Acemmanan in the Treatment of Recurrent Aphthous Stomatitis." *Wounds* 6 (1994): 40–45.

Mellon, Margaret. Press briefing on antibiotic resistance: causes and cures. Statement presented to the National Press Club, Washington, D.C., June 4, 1999.

Privitera, J. R. *Olive Leaf Extract: A New/Old Healing Bonanza for Mankind.* Covina, CA: Nutriscreen, 1966.

Pugliese, P., with J. Heinerman. *Devour Disease with Shark Liver Oil.* Green Bay, WI: Impakt Communications, 1999.

Pugliese, P., K. Jordan, and H. Cederberg. "Some Biological Actions of Alkylglycerols from Shark Liver Oil." *Journal of Alternative and Complementary Medicine.* 1: 87–99.

Regelson, W., R. Loria, and M. Kalimi. "Dehydroepiandrosterone (DHEA), the Mother Steroid. 1. Immunologic Action." *Annals of the New York Academy of Sciences* 719 (1994): 553–63.

Rice-Evans, C., and L. Packer. *Flavonoids in Health and Disease.* New York: Marcel Dekker, 1997.

Rittenhouse, J. R., Paul D. Lui, and Benjamin Lau. "Chinese Medicinal Herbs Reverse Macrophage Suppression Induced by Urological Tumors." *Journal of Urology* 146 (1991): 486–90.

Roberts, Robert. "N-acetylcysteine Enhances Antibody-Dependent Cellular Cytotoxicity in Neutrophils and Mononuclear Cells from Healthy Adults and Human Immunodeficiency Virus–Infected Patients." *Journal of Infectious Diseases* 172 (1995): 1492–1502.

Roebothan, B. V., and R. K. Chandra. "Relationships Between Nutritional Status and Immune Function of Elderly People." *Age and Aging* 23 (1994): 49–53.

Rountree, Robert. "The Herb-Drug Mix." *Herbs for Health,* July/August 1999, pp. 52–54.

———. "Protect Yourself from Colds and Flus." *Let's Live,* December 1998, pp. 61–64.

Santos, M., M. J. Gaziano, L. Leka, et al. "B-carotene-induced Enhancement of Natural Killer Cell Activity in Elderly Men: An Investigation of the Role of Cytokines." *American Journal of Clinical Nutrition* 68 (1998): 164–70.

Sapolsky, Robert M. *Why Zebras Don't Get Ulcers.* New York: W. H. Freeman and Co., 1994.

Schempp, C. M., K. Pelz, A. Wittmer, et al. "Antibacterial Activity of Hyperforin from St. John's Wort Against Multiresistant Staphylococcus Aureus and Gram-Positive Activity." *The Lancet,* June 19, 1999, p. 2129.

Schmidt, D. R. and A. E. Sabota. "An Examination of the Anti-Adherence Activity of Cranberry Juice on Urinary and Non-Urinary Bacterial Isolates." *Microbios* 55 (1988): 173.

Shahani, K. M., and A. Ayebo. "Role of Dietary Lactobacilli in Gastrointestinal Microecology." *American Journal of Clinical Nutrition* 33 (1980): 2448–57.

Shahani, K. M., J. R. Vakil, and A. Kilara. "Natural Antibiotic Activity of Lactobacillus Acidophilus and Bulgaricus." *Cultured Dairy Products Journal,* May 1977, pp. 8–11.

Shamsuddin, A. *IP6.* New York: Kensington Books, 1998.

Shamsuddin, A., and Guang-Yu Yang. "Inositol Hexaphosphate Inhibits Growth and Induces Differentiation of PC-3 Human Prostate Cancer Cells." *Carcinogensis* 16: 1975–79.

Shirota, M. "What You Should Know About Medicine Mushrooms." *Explore!* 7 (1996): 48–49.

Siciliano, A. "Cranberry." *Herbalgram* 38: 51–53.

Simopoulos, A. "Omega-3 Fatty Acids in Health and Disease and in Growth and Development." *American Journal of Clinical Nutrition* 54 (1991): 438–63.

Spake, A. "Losing the Battle of the Bugs." *U.S. News and World Report* 126: 52–60.

Stansbury, J. E. "Cancer Prevention Diet." *Nutrition Science News* 6 (1999): 382–86.

Stolberg, Sheryl G. "Superbugs: The Bacteria Antibiotics Can't Kill." *New York Times Magazine,* August 2, 1996, section 6, pp. 42–47.

"Study Only Confirms Echinacea Shouldn't Be Used as a Preventitive." *Prescription for Health,* July 1999.

"Thymic Protein A: Its Development May Signal a New Tool for Rejuvenating Immune Function." *Life Extension,* July 1997, pp. 21–25.

Tassou, C. C., and G. J. E. Nychas. "Inhibition of Salmonella Enteritidis by Oleuropein in Broth and in a Model Food System." *Letters in Applied Microbiology* 20 (1995): 120–24.

Tassou, C. C., G. J. E. Nychas, and R. G. Board. "Effect of Phenolic Compounds and Oleuropein on the Germination of *Bacillus cereus T* Spores." *Biotechnology and Applied Biochemistry* 13 (1991): 231–37.

Van Zandwijk, N. "N-acetylcysteine (NAC) and Glutathione (GSH): Antioxidant and Chemoprotective Properties, with Special Reference to Lung Cancer." *Journal of Cellular Biochemistry Supplement* 22 (1995): 24–32.

VERIS Research Summary. "The Protective Role of Antioxidants in the Aging Process." La Grange, IL: Veris Research Information Service, 1999.

Vojdani, A. "Natural Killer Cytotoxicity, Apoptosis and Cell

Cycle in Human Health and Diseases." Beverly Hills: Immunosciences Lab., Inc., 1997.

Vojdani, A., and M. Ghoneum. "In Vivo Effect of Ascorbic
Acid on Enhancement of Human Natural Killer Cell Activity." *Nutrition Research* 13 (1993): 753–64.

Walker, M. *Olive Leaf Extract.* New York: Kensington Pub-
lishing Group, 1997.

Weisberger, J. H. "Tea and Health: A Historical Perspective." *Cancer Letters* 114 (1997): 315–17.

Weisberger, J. H., and G. M. Williams. "Causes of Cancer."
In *American Cancer Society Textbook of Clinical Oncology,* edited
by G. P. Murphy, W. Lawrence, Jr., and R. Lenhard, Jr. 2nd
ed. Atlanta: American Cancer Society, 1995.

Whitaker, J. "Give Your Immune Cells a Natural 'Shot in
the Arm.'" *Health and Healing* 7 (1997): 1–2.

White, L. "Recovering from Surgery: Herbs That Heal."
*Nutrition Science News* 3 (1998): 316–20.

Whiteside, T., and R. Herberman. "Human Natural Killer
Cells in Health and Disease." *Clinical Immunotherapy* 1
(1994): 56–66.

Woodall, A. A., and B. N. Ames. "Diet and Oxidative Damage to DNA: The Importance of Ascorbate as an Antioxidant." In *Vitamin C in Health and Disease,* edited by L. Packer
and J. Fuchs. New York: Marcel Dekker, 1997.

Yang, C. S., and Z. W. Wang. "Tea and Cancer." *Journal of
the National Cancer Institute* 85: 1038–49.

Zakay-Rones, Z., N. Varsano, M. Zlotnick, et al. "Inhibition
of Several Strains of Influenza Virus in Vitro and Reduction
of Symptoms by an Elderberry Extract *(Sambucus nigra L.)*
During an Outbreak of Influenza B. Panama." *Journal of Alternative and Complementary Medicine* 1 (1995): 361–69.

Zand, J., R. Walton, and B. Rountree. *Smart Medicine for a Healthier Child.* Garden City, NY: Avery, 1994.

Zhao, K. S., C. Mancini, and G. Doria. "Enhancement of the Immune Response in Mice by *Astragalus membranaceus* Extracts." *Immunopharmacology* 20 (1990): 225–34.

Ziegler, R. G. "Vegetables, Fruits and Carotenoids and the Risk of Cancer." *American Journal of Clinical Nutrition* 53 (1991): 251S–59S.

Zimmerman, Marcia. "Immune Enhancers." *Nutrition Science News* 4 (1999): 84–90.

# Index

# About the Authors

## Robert Rountree, M.D.

Dr. Robert Rountree received his medical degree from the University of North Carolina School of Medicine at Chapel Hill in 1980. He subsequently completed a three-year residency in family and community medicine at the Milton S. Hershey Medical Center in Hershey, Pennsylvania, after which he was certified by the American Board of Family Practice.

Dr. Rountree has been providing his unique combination of traditional family medicine, nutrition, herbology, and mind-body therapy in Boulder, Colorado, since 1983. He currently practices at Helios Health Center, a multidisciplinary holistic clinic that he cofounded in 1993.

He is a coauthor of *Smart Medicine for a Healthier Child* (Avery, 1994) and *A Parent's Guide to Medical Emergencies*

(Avery, 1997), which integrate conventional medicine with herbal, nutritional, and other complementary approaches to children's health. He is also a featured subject in *An Alternative Medicine Definitive Guide to Cancer* (Future Medicine, 1997). His articles have appeared in *Herbs for Health, Let's Live,* and *Great Life* magazines.

In addition to lecturing widely and cohosting the radio program *Smart Medicine Radio* on KWAB-AM 1490 (http://www.radioforchange.com) in Boulder, Dr. Rountree is an assistant clinical professor in the department of family medicine at the University of Colorado School of Medicine. He serves on the advisory board for the Herb Research Foundation as well as the editorial boards of *The Journal of Alternative and Complementary Medicine, Nutrition Science News,* and *Delicious!* magazine. A member of the Wilderness Medical Society, he is passionate about the outdoors and enjoys hiking, backpacking, mountain biking, scuba diving, and world travel.

Early in his studies, he became deeply interested in a "patient-centered" approach to health and healing. Instead of following rigid protocols prescribed for specific diseases, he focused on the unique biochemical and emotional needs of individuals. To that end he has augmented his training with extensive postgraduate studies in nutritional and herbal pharmacology and with certification as a master practitioner of neurolinguistic programming.

## Carol Colman

Carol Colman is the *New York Times*–bestselling coauthor of *The Melatonin Miracle, Shed 10 Years in 10 Weeks,* and *Stop Depression Now,* among other successful books. She lives in Larchmont, New York, with her family.